SpringerBriefs in Modern Perspectives on Disability Research

Series Editors

Gabriel Bennett, Independent Researcher, Klemzig, Australia

Emma Goodall, Healthy Possibilities, Seaford, Australia

This book series on disability research is a comprehensive collection of research on disability and related issues. The series is designed to promote interdisciplinary collaboration and exchange, bringing together scholars and practitioners from different fields to share their perspectives and insights. Disability research is an interdisciplinary field that examines the social, cultural, historical, and political dimensions of disability. It encompasses a wide range of topics, including disability rights, accessibility, assistive technologies, healthcare, education, employment, and social welfare. Disability research scholars employ a range of theoretical and methodological approaches to understand the experiences of people with disabilities, as well as the ways in which disability intersects with other social identities such as race, gender, sexuality, and class.

The series seeks to advance knowledge and understanding of disability by publishing rigorous, innovative, and relevant research. It aims to promote disability rights and social justice by highlighting the ways in which people with disabilities are marginalized and discriminated against in society, and advocating for greater social inclusion and accessibility. The series also seeks to inform policy and practice by disseminating research findings that can help to shape policy decisions and contribute to positive social change.

Sheena Mariam Thomas ·
Ramakrishnan Veerabathiran

Disability and Decolonial Thought in Latin America

Indigenous Knowledge and Social Justice

Springer

Sheena Mariam Thomas
Human Cytogenetics and Genomics Laboratory, Faculty of Allied Health Sciences
Chettinad Hospital and Research Institute, Chettinad Academy of Research and Education
Kelambakkam, Tamil Nadu, India

Ramakrishnan Veerabathiran
Human Cytogenetics and Genomics Laboratory, Faculty of Allied Health Sciences
Chettinad Hospital and Research Institute, Chettinad Academy of Research and Education
Kelambakkam, Tamil Nadu, India

ISSN 3004-9709 ISSN 3004-9717 (electronic)
SpringerBriefs in Modern Perspectives on Disability Research
ISBN 978-981-95-8949-4 ISBN 978-981-95-8950-0 (eBook)
https://doi.org/10.1007/978-981-95-8950-0

This Springer imprint is published by the registered company Springer Nature Singapore Pte Ltd.
The registered company address is: 152 Beach Road, #21-01/04 Gateway East, Singapore 189721, Singapore

Preface

Disability has historically been considered through Eurocentric, biomedical, and rights-based approaches that proclaimed their universal nature while isolating others with different knowledge, being, and living with bodily and cognitive differences. In Latin America, the prevailing concepts have often fallen short of recognizing the uniqueness of the region's colonial pasts, racial stratification, Indigenous ways of thinking, and sociopolitical conflicts. The book, *Disability and Decolonial Thought in Latin America: Indigenous Knowledge and Social Justice*, is based on the belief that the issue of disability is inseparable from that of coloniality and that, on the contrary, the latter's end ceases to be a matter of whose lives are valued and whose suffering is normalized, the epistemologies that define the supreme justice to be served must be decolonized.

These chapters together present the case that in Latin America, disability is not only a medical or legal issue but rather a phenomenon that has been produced historically and is relationally dependent on colonial medicine, racial capitalism, land dispossession, forced assimilation, gender violence, and epistemic injustice. This has been the case from the very beginning, when colonial medical regimes were imposed that treated bodily differences as illnesses, to the present-day policy frameworks that acknowledge rights without offering actual justice in people's lives; disability has always been linked very closely to power structures that still control bodies, knowledge, and who belongs where.

This book unites decolonial disability studies, Indigenous worldviews, feminist theory, and grassroots activism to openly question and challenge such dominant narratives. It purposely redirects the perspective from the Global North to Latin America as a place not only of critical theory but also of resistance and the future alternatives. Indigenous ideas like relationality, reciprocity, collective care, and pluriversality are treated not as just supplementary views but rather as the very central epistemological foundations for the rethinking of disability itself. The book, therefore, resists the very inclination of making Western models of inclusion universal and instead brings to the forefront the meanings of justice that are locally grounded, culturally situated, and community-defined.

Every chapter has a part in achieving this supreme purpose by discussing disability in relation to colonial medicine and its legacies, racialization and epistemic exclusion, Indigenous ontologies of embodiment and care, land, territory and environmental violence, decolonial and Indigenous disability activisms, justice-oriented frameworks that go beyond rights-based inclusion, and grassroots policy knowledge coming from "below." All these chapters combined point to the fact that the issue of disability justice in Latin America is intertwined with the larger battles for Indigenous sovereignty, racial justice, gender justice, environmental justice, and decolonization.

This book is not about glorifying Indigenous peoples and communities nor portraying a decolonization process as a hassle-free solution. It is rather conducting a strong engagement with the prevailing internal contradictions, policy issues, and the problems associated with dealing with international legal frameworks, government bodies, and NGOs. The book acknowledges that the struggle for decolonial disability praxis continues, is contested, and is a collective process that necessitates being aware of and thinking through in ethical terms, being accountable, and having continuous discussions over it.

The manuscript is aimed at scholars, students, activists, policymakers, and practitioners who are involved in or interested in disability studies, Latin American studies, Indigenous studies, sociology, anthropology, public policy, and human rights, among others. It is, moreover, written in solidarity with the disabled Indigenous peoples and the grassroots movements who have been cut off from academic discourse far too often, and whose knowledge, struggles, and visions for the future have been disregarded.

Ultimately, the text expounds upon the decolonial thought in Latin America and disability that unavoidably asks for a fundamental shift of paradigm—from inclusion to justice, from universality to pluriversality, and from colonial categories of deficit to relational understandings of human difference. It opens a door for the readers to depict the future, where disability is not dictated by productivity, normalization, or charity, but instead rooted in care, interdependence, dignity, and collective responsibility.

Chennai, Tamil Nadu, India Sheena Mariam Thomas
January 2026 Ramakrishnan Veerabathiran

Acknowledgments The authors thank the Chettinad Academy of Research and Education for their constant support and encouragement.

Competing Interests The authors have no competing interests to declare that are relevant to the content of this manuscript.

About This Book

This book offers a groundbreaking examination of disability through the lens of decolonial theory and Indigenous epistemologies in Latin America. Challenging dominant Western biomedical and rights-based models, the volume foregrounds Indigenous worldviews, relational ontologies, and community-based understandings of embodiment, care, and inclusion. It explores how colonial legacies continue to shape structural marginalization, while also highlighting resistance, resilience, and cultural resurgence led by disabled Indigenous peoples and grassroots movements.

Through interdisciplinary analysis spanning anthropology, disability studies, Latin American studies, and political theory, the book critically interrogates how disability is constructed, represented, and addressed across diverse sociopolitical landscapes. Drawing on ethnographic accounts, oral histories, and community-driven initiatives, it provides a rich account of how Indigenous frameworks offer transformative possibilities for reclaiming dignity, autonomy, and justice. This work is a timely and essential contribution for scholars, practitioners, and activists interested in decolonial approaches to disability, intersectionality, and the reimagining of inclusive futures in the Global South.

Contents

Abbreviations

Afro-desc	Afro-descendant
BIPOC	Black, Indigenous, and People of Color
COVID-19	Coronavirus Disease 2019
CRPD	Convention on the Rights of Persons with Disabilities
CSR	Corporate Social Responsibility
DDR	Disability Rights Movement
DJM	Disability Justice Movement
DJS	Disability Justice Studies
DS	Disability Studies
EDI	Equity, Diversity, and Inclusion
EJ	Environmental Justice
GN	Global North
GS	Global South
ICHR	International Convention on Human Rights
INGO	International Non-Governmental Organization
IP	Indigenous Peoples
LA	Latin America
LAC	Latin America and the Caribbean
LGBTQ+	Lesbian, Gay, Bisexual, Transgender, Queer/Questioning, and Others
NEP	Neoliberal Economic Policies
NGO	Non-Governmental Organization
PWD / PwD	Persons with Disabilities
SAPs	Structural Adjustment Programs
SDGs	Sustainable Development Goals
SSD	South–South Dialogue
SSM	South–South Movements
STEM	Science, Technology, Engineering, and Mathematics
UDHR	Universal Declaration of Human Rights
UN	United Nations
UNDP	United Nations Development Programme

UNESCO	United Nations Educational, Scientific and Cultural Organization
WHO	World Health Organization

List of Figures

List of Tables

Chapter 1
Colonial Medicine and the Making of the Disabled Body

Abstract The focus of this chapter is on showing that disability in things happened as a result of colonial medicine in Latin America rather than merely as a result of biological impairment. To support its argument, the chapter draws on decolonial disability studies and asserts that colonial medical regimes, through their power to define Indigenous, Afro-descendant, and colonized bodies as sick, helped imperial governance, capitalist extraction, and racial hierarchies. Under the pretext of a "civilizing mission," Western biomedicine, which was introduced, displaced holistic Indigenous health systems that stressed balance, spirituality, communal care, and body diversity. Colonial medicine applied racial science, asylums, eugenics, and labor-based classification of bodily "fitness" as mechanisms to turn difference into deficit and thereby legitimize segregation, surveillance, and coercion. The chapter shows how disability was closely connected to coloniality, and how modern ideas of normalcy, productivity, and health originated together with capitalism and European epistemological control. The paper also points out the differences between these impositions and pre-colonial Indigenous worldviews that acknowledged different bodies as necessary for the community and that placed people in other social roles by means of reciprocity rather than exclusion. The dissection of the past further reveals that colonial violence, in its various forms such as forced labor, displacement, epidemics, environmental degradation, and reproductive control, not only caused impairment directly but also, by medicalizing suffering, denied people access to the structural sources of their suffering. Emphasizing the resistance of Indigenous peoples, the plurality of medical practices, and the involvement of the community in healthcare, the chapter reveals the persistence of alternative ways of knowing even under colonial imposition. In the end, the author argues that to understand the present-day disability inequalities in Latin America, one has to consider the lasting impacts of colonial medicine. Thus, a decolonial angle on disability is necessary not only for regaining power and rewriting historical narratives but also for envisioning future societies that are fairer and more inclusive, thus having their roots in the customary wisdom and practical experience of the people.

Keywords Colonial medicine · Disability studies · Decolonial theory · Indigenous health · Latin America

S. M. Thomas and R. Veerabathiran, *Disability and Decolonial Thought in Latin America*, SpringerBriefs in Modern Perspectives on Disability Research,
https://doi.org/10.1007/978-981-95-8950-0_1

1.1 Introduction

The colonial histories in Latin America have profoundly affected the understanding and experience of disability, where the colonial project and medical authority primarily played a role in creating disability as a category under the empire. This viewpoint supports the notion that disability is not just an inherent biological problem but a very dynamic social and political phenomenon that is very closely linked to historical power relations and systemic inequalities. The decolonial perspectives in disability studies are the ones that provide the most emphasis on the necessity of going against Eurocentric presumptions that have been the very foundation of the field, and through this, acknowledging that traditional Western conceptions are the ones who universalize experiences and the ones who neglect different cultural, historical, and geopolitical contexts (Chaves, 2022; Dirth & Adams, 2019; Ferrari, 2020; Grech, 2017; Lapierre, 2023; Meekosha, 2011; Ortega, 2023; Roy, 2024).

The colonial endeavor greatly affected the disability perception, classification, and management of disabilities in Latin America. Rather than a neutral science, colonial medicine was a very powerful instrument of control, which was used to manage populations, extract wealth, and enforce hierarchies. The very instrumental role of medicine meant that the power to define disease became merged with the power to control people, especially in colonial settings (Brieger, 2004; Seaton, 2020). The bodies of the colonized populations were sometimes regarded as economic resources to be managed for profit, especially in the case of labor-intensive contexts such as plantations (Lapierre, 2023). This viewpoint is consistent with bioplastics, where controlling populations means managing their collective biological life: health, birth rates, hygiene, and longevity as a political and economic resource (Mignolo, 2000).

Disability was, in this colonial context, quite often viewed through the lens of the medical model and subjected to segregation, thus determining the individuals according to their "fitness" for work. In stark contrast to this, a number of native systems of health care were much more humane, and their concerned methods were focused mainly on the individual's social integration, reciprocity, and finding flexible community roles for them regardless of their ability. For example, the indigenous communities in Latin America, besides being fully aware of the disability imposed by colonization, developed their own worldviews and cultural practices through which they understood and experienced the disability. Moreover, the economic and social conditions of and political violence against these indigenous communities that are the result of colonial power relations are the main factors that further contribute to the disability of such populations (Hernández et al., 2024; Lapierre, 2023).

Coloniality as a concept denotes the survival of the colonial period hierarchies in the forms of power, resource, and knowledge distribution, even after the disappearance of the political entities (Dirth & Adams, 2019; Goikolea-Amiano, 2020; Harding, 2016). The decolonial theory in Latin America posits that the whole of modernity, its politics and epistemology, is seen more clearly if the viewpoint of the colonized people of the Americas, by Spanish and Portuguese, is taken into consideration (Harding, 2016; Mignolo, 2000). This theory shows that the trio of European colonialism, modernity, and capitalism is ambiguously intertwined; the very definition of knowledge and skill was shaped by their interaction (Dirth & Adams, 2019; Goikolea-Amiano, 2020; Harding, 2016).

The colonizers often equated norms for the human body with being productive and racial ranking, which ultimately worked in favor of the existing system of discrimination against disabled people and persecution of those with disabilities (Setio, 2026). One of the areas where this is best illustrated is research done in some regions of Latin America concerning the extent of intellectual disabilities, which reports a higher rate due to causative agents like malnutrition, lack of perinatal care, and contamination with toxic and infectious agents, all of which are more prevalent in the poorest regions of the world that are often the remnant of colonial economies (Mercadante et al., 2009). In addition to these causative factors, the past had diseases such as goiter and cretinism, where people might have been judged living in social oppression and neocolonialism in countries like El Salvador (Vrana, 2023). Accounts of leprosy in Peru tell a historical story that even includes possible pre-Hispanic references, and thus one can see how such diseases were considered and combated in the course of centuries (Ashmead, 1894; Ashmead, 1895).

The colonial-era asylum is a prime example of how the disability issue was managed across the empire. These medical institutions usually acted like both clinics and prisons, with most of the patients being those sent by the police or who were working as inmates. Racial science was used frequently as the basis for diagnoses, and new categories were created that classified indigenous peoples as sick. The main aim was not to heal the person in a modern way but to lock up those who were regarded as unproductive or disturbing to the public order. The same thinking is found in the methods used by colonial medicine, which often practiced the medicalization of disability and its segregation, along with defining people by their "fitness" for labor (Lapierre, 2023).

It is essential to differentiate impairment (a bodily difference) from disability (the social disadvantage that results from society not accommodating that impairment) at this point (González-Calle et al., 2023; Javier et al., 2013; Summerhill, 1800). The social model of disability, which goes against the traditional medical model, claims that disability is caused by barriers erected by society and not by the individual impairments (Boveda et al., 2019). This model has passed on to the disability rights movements in Latin America, where the activism that takes place is mainly centered on recognition and political influence, supported by legislative frameworks like the Convention on the Rights of Persons with Disabilities (Brégain et al., 2022; Rebolledo-Sanhueza & Galaz-Valderrama, 2024). Nonetheless, even if the situation has improved, there are still major implementation bottlenecks that have to be dealt with (Rebolledo-Sanhueza & Galaz-Valderrama, 2024).

In Latin America, the decolonization of disability studies and practices, which is a very active movement, is questioning the Eurocentric views and trying to connect disability with the indigenous peoples' understanding (Ferrari, 2020; Lapierre, 2023; Ortega, 2023; Roy, 2024). This involves turning the concept of disability upside down, accepting non-normative bodies, and creating alternative responses to colonial ontologies. For instance, decolonial feminisms offer the analytical categories that allow us to critically examine the definitions of disability in the Latin American context and to propose new frameworks with points of intersection around disability issues. Also, research indicates that cultural competence should be integrated into health systems, particularly in relation to the understanding of suffering that falls outside Western diagnostic categories and the existence of linguistic barriers for indigenous peoples. A decolonial viewpoint that acknowledges the historical dominance of the medical profession and the construction of disability as a category to serve imperial purposes is crucial for the understanding of disability in Latin America (Ferrari, 2020; Ortega, 2023; Roy, 2024). This new way of thinking demands a thorough investigation into how much past colonial practices still play a crucial role in the shaping of present-day policies, public perceptions, and the lives of disabled people in the region (Grech, 2017; Meekosha, 2011; Setio, 2026).

1.2 Pre-colonial Indigenous Conceptions on Health, Body, and Difference

Pre-colonial indigenous views on health, the human body, and even differences among disabled individuals in Latin America were profoundly influenced by cosmologies that see well-being as holistic, community care systems, spiritual healing practices, and an innate perception of body diversity and social membership (Lapierre, 2023; Lovern, 2017; Stienstra & Ashcroft, 2010; Weaver, 2015). These views are in stark contrast to the Western biomedical models, which typically consider disability as a personal deficit that needs healing (Schleck & Ben-Alon, 2024; Zaks, 2024). However, indigenous worldviews focus on the interconnectedness of lives, the collective well-being, and the different facets of health, including physical, spiritual, and social ones being integrated (Janka et al., 2024; Rosales-Rivadeneira et al., 2017; Stienstra & Ashcroft, 2010).

Indigenous people from Latin America are able to interpret and live disability in their own specific and cultural ways, which are often at the same time with realities of disability that are made worse by colonialism, assimilation, and poor socio-economic conditions (Lapierre, 2023). The colonial encounter with its political, social, economic, and cultural implications has been a disabling and devastating factor to indigenous populations, often leading to epistemic injustices where indigenous viewpoints are marginalized or misinterpreted (Devakumar et al., 2022; Grech, 2017; Meekosha, 2011).

Holistic Cosmologies of Well-being: The cosmologies of indigenous people in Latin America naturally associate health and illness with the universe's various aspects, where the spiritual, environmental, and social factors are tightly linked to an individual's well-being (Rosales-Rivadeneira et al., 2017; Stienstra & Ashcroft, 2010). The state of being healthy is seen as one of harmony and balance, and the disturbances in this balance can appear as sickness or being disabled, or sometimes even just being disabled in one's own perception (Rosales-Rivadeneira et al., 2017;

Weaver, 2015). To give an example, the Otavalo community in Ecuador accepts health and sickness through the lens of an intercultural Andean viewpoint, stressing the use of plants along with other traditional methods to heal both the body and the mind (Rosales-Rivadeneira et al., 2017).

The body, in many indigenous belief systems, is not just a biological entity but is closely tied to kin, community, and the cosmos (Lara, 2008; Rodríguez, 2020). This relational view of the world and existence is one of the main reasons why practices like curanderismo have been and still are developed; a system of healing based on the belief that health is a harmony between body, spirit, community, and nature, has its roots in Latin America (Schmidt, 2021). Healing rituals, herbal pharmacology, and the "meaning response" are all the inherent features of this holistic approach, where the context and belief surrounding a treatment can have tangible physiological effects (Brueggemann & Ekwonye, 2023; Schmidt, 2021). The effectiveness of indigenous healing rituals can be explained by psychobiological mechanisms that relieve pain and stress, the endogenous opioid release, and the support of the community.

Mental health issues, for example, are very often interpreted in terms of "spiritual disharmonies" which may be caused by and are combined with the aforementioned factors like territorial displacement, loss of language, and a disconnect from cultural competence in healthcare systems. The Emberá Dobida community in Colombia, for example, has to deal with a spiritual crisis in its midst that is causing the most significant and most terrible loss of their territory and the problem of communication, and thus, their external factors are significantly affecting their internal well-being (Hernández et al., 2024).

Communal Care Systems and Spiritual Healing: The indigenous societies mainly rely on communal care systems for their support and daily living, which is a colossal net of mutual responsibility for everyone's wellness (Weaver, 2015). Such systems frequently consist of interconnectedness via family, kinship, and community (Crocetti et al., 2024). In such situations, the care of persons with disabilities becomes a matter of society as a whole instead of the specialized, usually isolating, institutions (Solsona-Cisternas, 2025). For instance, in many indigenous cultures, if a person has a "disability" or difference, they are kept in a community, their role and responsibility are emphasized, which eventually leads to a feeling of belonging and contribution (Weaver, 2015).

Spiritual healing is considered by many to be the mainstay of these care systems, and it is the one that provides ways to deal with not only physical but also mental and spiritual ailments (Brueggemann & Ekwonye, 2023; Lara, 2008; Schmidt, 2021). A number of different spiritual healing practices have been derived from indigenous peoples' customs and are practiced in the Latin American region, such as in Mexico and Peru (Schmidt, 2021). The practices usually involve those healers who connect with the native beliefs and then apply various rituals, prayers, and natural remedies in order to achieve the desired state of health (Lara, 2008; Rosales-Rivadeneira et al., 2017; Schmidt, 2021). The study of Latina health activist-healers, for example, reveals how the indigenous-inspired viewpoints are countering the Western conception of the body/spirit dichotomy and, at the same time, sexuality and spirituality are being integrated into the healing process (Lara, 2008).

The incorporation of spiritual practices into health is even seen in modern healthcare settings. In Brazil, the indigenous spirituality causes difficulties for the health specialists in the case of treating children's chronic diseases, which makes it clear that intercultural communication and sharing of traditional healing methods are to be developed (de Freitas et al., 2023). The "Buen Vivir" plan in Ecuador is intended to combine ancestral medical knowledge and the experiences of traditional healers with formal health services, which is a sign of the worldview acceptance of these practices (Bautista-Valarezo et al., 2021).

In some West African tribes, the pre-colonial reasoning viewed those persons whom the Western world regarded as "disabled" as having special powers; thus, the social ethos, healing practices, and folklore became the arenas where such differences were positively perceived. This view was sometimes still in place among the enslaved peoples of the Americas, which is an indication of the cultural interconnections that were maintained (Barclay, 2017).

Body Diversity and Social Belonging: Indigenous cultures have generally accepted body diversity as an inherent aspect of humans, often opposing the Western notion of disability (Lovern, 2017, 2022). In the past, disability was not necessarily equated with "disability" in the Western context but was more like a difference or an alternative way of being (Senier, 2013). This very acceptance encourages social belonging; individuals with diverse abilities are accepted in the community and work according to their strengths (Weaver, 2015).

The notion of "inappropriated bodies" posited in Southern Latin American cities shows how the meaning of death is related to bodies, thus the embodiment of disability through social conditions (Rodríguez, 2020). This demonstrates the role of social and cultural contexts in determining the views of the body and its variations.

Nonetheless, the enforcement of colonial paradigms has brought in Western medical models that regard differences as diseases, which often culminate in the same negative consequences of stigma and exclusion that were non-existent in the pre-colonial period with respect to indigenous perceptions of (Grech, 2017; Lapierre, 2023; Weaver, 2015; Zaks, 2024). The advocates for the decolonization of point out the necessity of adopting indigenous viewpoints as one way to counteract Eurocentric understandings, and thus, opening the way for more inclusive (Grech, 2017; Meekosha, 2011; Puszka et al., 2022). This further implies that we should acknowledge the distinctive situations of the disabled indigenous people and their non-involvement in the Western disability debates (Velarde, 2018).

In Colombia, the terms aidaiza and baa wa wa/jai wa wa from the Murui Muina-Minika and Êbêra Eyábida indigenous worlds, respectively, refer to the same matter but through different linguistic forms that are not so Western dependent (Chan et al., 2023; Yarza de los Ríos, 2020). The indigenous meanings behind these words express different kinds of the two worlds' visions (anthropoecogenic and theoecogenic), thus indicating different ways of looking at the issue of diversity, which are very important for coming up with expressions around the whole issue of body diversity. The ongoing effects of colonialism and the dominance of the global North in disability studies have often led to the marginalization of the experiences of the global South, thereby causing an "intellectual crisis" for disability studies in these regions (Connell, 2011;

Meekosha, 2011). Decolonizing disability studies involves a radical rethinking of concepts, the interpretation of disability as a result of colonial violence, capitalist accumulation, and hierarchical gender relations (Connell, 2011).

The pre-Columbian indigenous concepts of health and disability among the disabled in Latin America repose in a holistic framework wherein health is a product of balance and interconnectedness, communal care systems render intrinsic and continuous support, and spiritual healing is accorded a crucial place in the treatment of illness and suffering. Such a framework is also supportive of body diversity, thus leading to a strong sense of belonging that has been weakened by the imposition of Western, ableist views through colonization (Connell, 2011; Lapierre, 2023; Lovern, 2017; Weaver, 2015). Knowing these indigenous viewpoints is essential for the promotion of health equality and decolonization of disability approaches (Chandanabhumma & Narasimhan, 2020; Puszka et al., 2022). Table 1.1 depicts the Indigenous Disability Activism in Latin America.

1.3 Colonial Medical Regimes and the Pathologization of Indigenous Bodies

The colonial medical regimes that were set up in Latin America and later on propagated Western biomedicine and scientific racialization through the clinics ultimately changed the understanding and experience of disability for the worse, mainly by the pathologizing of the Indigenous bodies (Hutcheon & Lashewicz, 2020; Lapierre, 2023; Ortega, 2023). Such a historical process, often connected with a "civilizing mission," redefined the concept of disability and its use as a means of control, thus strengthening social order through the reinforcement of hierarchies and justifications for the exploitation of the marginalized (Grech, 2017; Hutcheon & Lashewicz, 2020; Lapierre, 2023).

The colonization of Latin America brought about the introduction of Western biomedicine, which in turn caused the encounter between the European and the Indigenous medical systems. The European colonizers would usually consider the Indigenous medical practices as superstitious and thus would impose their own biomedical framework over them. The whole scenario was sometimes referred to as the first era of medical pluralism, where Hispanic medicine was laid over the already existing Indian medical systems (Menéndez, 2015; Newson, 2006; Sowell, 2003). This, however, was not a mere swapping of practices but rather a taking over of Indigenous medical knowledge, for example, the use of quinine, without giving proper credit, thus reinforcing the imperial hierarchies (Fredrick, 2021). The explorer-anthropologists would often go through regions like Patagonia and Pampas, having very little medical training, and would diagnose, treat, and at times even "cure" the Indigenous people, publishing their observations in hybrid travelogue-ethnographies (Kerr, 2020). This marked a significant turning point wherein Western

Table 1.1 Indigenous disability activism in Latin America—actors, practices, and decolonial contributions

Dimension of activism	Specific features in indigenous disability activism	Key practices and strategies	Political and epistemic significance	Representative studies
Intersectional foundations	Activism rooted in indigenous identity, disability experience, gender, class, and colonial history	Collective organizing across indigenous, feminist, and disability movements	Challenges single-axis disability frameworks; foregrounds lived intersectionality	Daniels-Mayes (2023), Meekosha (2011)
Reivindicative political practices	Demand for recognition as political subjects rather than welfare recipients	Public demonstrations, community assemblies, advocacy within indigenous councils	Repositions disability as a political identity linked to indigenous sovereignty	Pino-Morán et al. (2023), Rebolledo-Sanhueza and Galaz-Valderrama (2024)
Community-based organizing	Activism embedded in communal life rather than individual leadership	Collective decision-making, kinship-based support systems	Resists neoliberal individualization of disability rights	Bachfischer et al. (2023)
Epistemic resistance	Rejection of biomedical dominance in defining disability	Use of indigenous languages, cosmologies, and oral histories	Produces counter-knowledge challenging Eurocentric disability theory	Grech (2017), Roy (2024)
Decolonial framing of disability	Disability understood as relational, social, and environmental	Reframing impairment as socially produced through colonial violence	Shifts disability analysis from pathology to structural injustice	Meekosha (2011), Lapierre (2023)
Indigenous healing and care as activism	Healing practices mobilized as political resistance	Community healing rituals, traditional medicine	Undermines colonial medical authority and segregation	Baez et al. (2024)
Gender-focused indigenous activism	Leadership of indigenous disabled women	Advocacy against reproductive violence and sterilization	Links disability activism to reproductive justice	Acevedo et al. (2023), Ferrari (2020)

(continued)

Table 1.1 (continued)

Dimension of activism	Specific features in indigenous disability activism	Key practices and strategies	Political and epistemic significance	Representative studies
Engagement with state institutions	Strategic participation in policy spaces without full assimilation	Policy consultations, legal advocacy	Exposes gaps between formal rights and lived realities	Pinilla-Roncancio (2015)
Critique of rights-based models	Skepticism toward universalized disability rights frameworks	Adaptation of rights discourse to indigenous contexts	Highlights cultural incommensurability of Western legal models	Grech (2017), Roy (2024)
Territorial and environmental activism	Disability linked to land dispossession and environmental harm	Protests against extractivism and pollution	Frames disability as a consequence of environmental racism	Rougeon et al. (2023)
Cultural expression as resistance	Use of art, ritual, storytelling	Cultural performances, collective memory work	Reclaims indigenous disabled bodies as knowledge holders	Pino-Morán et al. (2023)
Transnational and regional networks	Collaboration across Latin America	Knowledge exchange and solidarity movements	Builds regional decolonial disability agendas	Daniels-Mayes (2023)
Policy impact and limitations	Partial influence on disability legislation	Local-level policy shifts rather than systemic change	Reveals structural resistance within state systems	Rebolledo-Sanhueza and Galaz-Valderrama (2024)
Disability as a site of resistance	Disability used to challenge colonial power relations	Activism beyond disability-specific demands	Positions disability within broader anti-colonial struggles	Meekosha (2011), Pino-Morán et al. (2023)

medicine began to show its power and, by medicalizing the local suffering, would often misinterpret the local people's experience of suffering (Menéndez, 2015).

Racialized science was a vital element in this whole process by introducing terms like "folie indigène" (native madness) in the colonial asylums that performed the dual role of hospitals and jails. The intention behind these establishments was often seclusion rather than healing, and the inmates were mainly those who were considered unproductive or disturbing. Scientific racism is an abuse of science, which applies scientific techniques to invent a false biological rank for the races, resulting in the labeling of rebels as sick and the application of "treatments" that are coercive by nature, being justified. One of the classic examples is the case of "drapetomania," a so-called mental disorder that caused the enslaved to run away, thus making the craving for liberation a sickness and the imprisonment of the slaves a medically approved action. This racialization also embraced the health issues, and diseases were usually portrayed in the light of "tropicality" or "native habits," thus hiding the fundamental social causes. The students' views regarding the cultural competence, medical culture, and racial bias in their profession are still shaped by a "white logic, white curriculum" that can conceptualize race and reinforce the medical hierarchies (Plaisime et al., 2023).

As part of the "civilizing mission," disease narratives were used in a very clever way to justify the colonial intervention and control over the Indigenous peoples (Carey Jr, 2019). Displacement of the Indian population through public health measures in colonial Latin America, as well as in other colonial areas, took place according to the economic and military interests rather than on the basis of humanitarian concerns. The colonized people's health was seen in terms of labor's maximum output and strength of military forces; hence, health was not the end but the means to economic plunder or military conquest. For example, the endemic goiter and cretinism in El Salvador were the issues of concern for public health researchers, but the very tools utilized to evaluate these conditions often failed to reveal the social and political inequalities and neocolonialism hidden beneath them (Vrana, 2023). This methodology used to be the basis for the enactment of public health measures like hospitals for the segregated population and mandatory quarantines that were directed at and had a disproportionately negative impact on the colonized populations. It was not just improvement in health that was the objective, but also maintaining a productive labor force and enforcing social order.

The act of mapping "abnormality" turned out to be a colonial practice where the colonizers determined disability to further their aims (Hutcheon & Lashewicz, 2020; Lapierre, 2023; Ortega, 2023). The disability among Latin American Indigenous peoples is both understood and experienced in accordance with their own worldview and cultural practices; however, these are at the same time coexisting with the disability produced by the colonial domination and enforced assimilation (Lapierre, 2023).

Disability during colonial times was seen in terms of medicalization and segregation, where people were categorized according to their "fitness" for labor. This was in stark contrast to the systems of many Indigenous communities, where the focus was on social integration and finding flexible roles within the community. The term "disability" can be considered as a colonial tool, particularly for the bodies that got labeled disabled; it had far-reaching implications in ontological and ethical-political domains (Ortega, 2023). The arrangement of authorities, resources, and knowledge in a colonial way that has lasted had been a significant determinant of how the people of the Global South perceive disabilities (Grech, 2017; Meekosha, 2011). For instance, research in Chile points to the existence of coloniality and its manifestation in the form of dominant medicine and traditional psychiatry, which are present in most Latin American countries. It also shows the subjective and social process of transforming one's identity in monopolistic groups like doctors, which is still going on in Latin America (Sepúlveda Jara & Oyarce Pisani, 2020).

Colonial dominions had control over the disability issue as a form of power through medical sciences. Medical classifications were employed to map the social ladder and hence make some groups invisible and subdued (Hutcheon & Lashewicz, 2020; Ortega, 2023). The application of Western diagnostic categories, at times leading to "category fallacy," disregarded the Indigenous people's concept of suffering as "idioms of distress," which are rooted in social and spiritual disharmonies. For instance, the Emberá Dobida people think of spiritual disharmonies in terms of suffering related to land, body, and language, which takes a toll on psychological well-being, especially among children and youth who have increased suicide rates. When a family loses its ancestral land, the chain of traditions associated with that land and the people's identity is broken, and hence they not only suffer physically but also emotionally and spiritually. This can lead to a state of un-Wellness that encompasses the whole family. In the same way, issues such as eating difficulties and sadness point out that the process of language acquisition is very much dependent on emotional and physical well-being. The lack of cultural understanding in health systems, especially when it comes to suffering outside the scope of Western diagnosis and the Spanish language, highlights the difficulties Indigenous communities are encountering (Hernández et al., 2024). The presence of disabled workers was considered a reason for the unfair treatment in the colonial labor market (Hutcheon & Lashewicz, 2020). The acceptance of biopolitical practices on plantations, for example, regarded the enslaved bodies as mere labor units, and medicine was concerned with their performance as a workforce rather than with their well-being as a goal in itself. This type of reasoning shaped the medical planning, where health became one of the factors in the calculations made to either maximize military effectiveness or economic output. The "iron law of democratic socialism" brings to light the rift between capitalism and democracy, with the former being the epitome of inequality and the latter the symbol of equality, thus revealing how economic systems can be the cause of social disparities and exploitation (Dale, 2014). The legal and practical disadvantages imposed on people with darker skin in colonial Latin America indicate the existence of caste-like hierarchies, which also reflect the attitudes and practices that supported labor exploitation (Grieshaber, 1979).

Missions, hospitals, and state institutions were crucial in the control of bodies and the imposition of colonial power (Boodman, 2023; Carey Jr, 2019). Medical practice in early colonial Spanish America was not solely through state institutions, but rather through the close cooperation of the state and the Church (Newson, 2006). Populations of disabled people were among those managed by these institutions. The colonial asylum, a cross between a clinic and a prison, was where persons considered to be non-productive or to disturb the peace were confined. Even today, medical colonialism is still an ongoing material relation, where settler care and Indigenous dispossession cannot be separated. This signifies that care and violence have a common ground, hence the need for a decolonial care ethic that will not only render powerless the colonizers' flow of care but also the counteracting power of the colonized (Boodman, 2023). The field of Physical Medicine and Rehabilitation (PM&R) in Latin America has been growing in the past 60 years, dealing with disability and restoring function. Nonetheless, disability is a greater hazard for women, older people, and ethnic minorities in low-income countries in Latin America (Schiappacasse et al., 2019).

Since the 1800s, the "medical model of disability," which is prevalent, perceives disabilities as deviances that are to be cured or eliminated, thus concentrating on the body's conforming to a "normal" ideal. The stress on normalization has been a significant disadvantage to disabled individuals (Zaks, 2024). The "social model," in contrast, claims that the leading cause of disability is not individual impairments but rather the barriers created by society, thereby changing the focus from fixing people to fixing the world. Critical disability studies and decolonial frameworks scrutinize the "coloniality of ability," successfully showing how the concept of disability has been historically constructed and deployed to support power asymmetries (Ferrari, 2020; Grech, 2017; Hutcheon & Lashewicz, 2020; Ortega, 2023). These frameworks not only dictate but also support the interpretations of disability that are inclusive and guided mainly by the voices and experiences of disabled people from the Global South (Meekosha, 2011; Woods et al., 2018).

1.4 Eugenics, Racial Hygiene, Adaptation, and the Latin American Context

Eugenics, racial hygiene, and their involvement with disability in Latin America create a complicated and ancient historical path that has an impact on the society's views, policies, and experiences of Indigenous, Afro-descendant, and mixed-race groups. The intellectual eugenics basis in Latin America can be traced back to the beginning of the twentieth century, when the nineteenth-century social Darwinism and positivism were discredited and reshaped by religion, nationalism, and international scientific exchange. Sanctioning a more subtle coercive environment, Latin American eugenicists often accepted neo-Lamarckian principles, which put the focus on environmental modification and areas like puericulture (infant and child hygiene) as a way to "improve" the population. Nevertheless, the racial hierarchy still continued to some extent, which was the case with Chile's eugenic nationalism that, while recognizing mestizaje, still held the view of racial superiority (de Souza et al., 2021; Lapierre, 2023; Stern, 2016; Walsh, 2019a, 2019b).

Adaptations of European Eugenics and the Targeting of Vulnerable Populations: In Latin America, the concept of eugenics was often associated with the medical rhetoric of "racial improvement" by public health, hygiene, and controlled reproduction, which was usually framed within a nationalist discourse of strengthening the nation (Stern, 2016; Walsh, 2019a). Brazil, for example, was one country where local eugenics movements led to the establishment of educational, vocational, and residential services for individuals with intellectual disabilities, which were similar to practices in the United States at that time (Block, 2007). These movements looked at the bodies of Indigenous, Afro-descendant, and mixed-race people as being sick by relating them to supposed intellectual or physical "defects," and thus legitimizing social control and discrimination (de Souza et al., 2021). Among others, such eugenic ideas helped to establish the marginalization and medicalization of disability in these groups through subtle, insidious ways, like public health campaigns rather than overt, legal mandates for sterilization, though prenuptial certificates were debated as a eugenic measure in some countries, such as Spain, which has implications for Latin American thought (Walin, 2023). The critiques of eugenics, both in the past and at present, point to the fact that its very fundamental premise was flawed, thereby bringing the whole notion of biological inferiority and the "menace" to the eugenicists' perception of disability into question (Linett, 2024). The medical model of disability, which sees disability as a problem located within the individual and assumes that it is possible to cure or prevent it, conforms to eugenic thinking by aiming at the elimination of all conditions classified as "defects."

Gender, Reproduction, and Colonial Control of Fertility: The control of fertility among women in particular became one of the main aspects of eugenic and colonial practices in Latin America (Bueno & Pardo, 2023). Disabled women, primarily Indigenous women and girls, have faced gender-based violence disproportionately, which very frequently overlaps with the issues of reproduction and bodily autonomy (Acevedo et al., 2023). The colonial control of fertility was imposed on the Indigenous and Afro-descendant women whose bodies were very often perceived through the prism of racial purity or national height, resulting in the implementation of policies and practices that were meant to regulate their reproductive choices (Franceschet & Thomas, 2016). This context of history brings to the present not only the issue of abortion but also the issue of fertility treatment, which is still considered a privilege among people experiencing poverty because of the societal perception of disabled people as vulnerable and too much risk to have children (Sanmiquel-Molinero et al., 2023).

Violence, Trauma, and the Production of Impairment: The colonial legacy in Latin America has a very close connection with the impairment caused by different types of violence and trauma.

Forced labor, displacement, and war: The colonial past and its structures still in place have caused forced labor and displacement, which in turn directly lead to disability (Angarita-Cañas, 2020). Political violence and socio-economic conditions are among the main reasons for the higher-than-average rate of disability among Indigenous groups (Lapierre, 2023). The colonized bodies were often seen as commodities, and their source of profit was primarily through the plantation system, where medicament was employed to not only keep the labor force but also fertilize the ground for profiting through their hiring out.

Epidemics introduced through colonization: The process of colonization was the cause of the introduction of new diseases to the native population, leading to the spread of epidemics that knocked down a large number of people and caused long-term disabilities and disabilities, thus changing demographics and health patterns (Ramos, 2021).

Environmental destruction and long-term disabling effects: Environmental racism, a term that is slowly gaining recognition in the context of Latin America and Brazil, shows that the Indigenous and Afro-descendant populations, who are already marginalized, suffer the most due to the ecological damage, the latter even being the result of pollution from factories intended to cause chronic health problems and thus, impairment (Meireles et al., 2018; Rougeon et al., 2023). The issue of a connection between the environment and health has a long history, such as the fear of goiter and its supposed connection to cretinism being recognized as inseparable from social inequality and neocolonialism (Sundberg, 2008; Vrana, 2023).

Indigenous Resistance, Healing, and Counter-Epistemologies: To counteract the systemic pressures, Indigenous societies in Latin America have developed strong resistance and healing practices.

Survival of traditional medicine: Traditional medicine, which embraces an all-encompassing concept of health, has its roots in history and continues to play a significant role in the cultural identity of Latin America. It is a medical alternative to biomedicine, especially in situations where the latter is socially rejected, or access is limited, or the costs are high (Baez et al., 2024).

Hybrid practices and medical pluralism: The meeting point of European and Indigenous medicine did not always lead to the total demise of the latter. Instead, intricate processes of syncretism came up, giving birth to hybrid medical practices that used Indigenous wisdom coupled with colonial medical techniques (Musante, 2019). Medical pluralism, the opportunity to use non-biomedical practices (like native American therapies, natural medicines, and complementary alternatives) in healthcare models, is a remarkable feature of the Latin American health systems, even though its regulation and conception are inconsistent among the different countries (Papalini & Avelín Cesco, 2022).

Community-led care as resistance to colonial categorization: Indigenous healing systems place a great emphasis on social integration, reciprocity, and very flexible community roles for people with various abilities, which is in stark contrast to colonial medicine that would label people with disabilities and separate them from the rest of society. Community-based inclusive development is a strategy adopted in Latin America to empower the rights of people with disabilities and to address their needs through community participation (Bachfischer et al., 2023). The community-led initiatives can be perceived as a type of resistance to the distortion of colonial medical narratives and their classifications of disability (Pino-Moran et al., 2023).

Decolonizing Disability: Reclaiming Agency and Rewriting Histories: To decolonize disability means to oppose the Eurocentric viewpoint that has dominated disability studies and to systematically reclaim the narratives and agency (Grech, 2017; Meekosha, 2011; Roy, 2024).

Challenging colonial medical narratives: The field of disability studies, particularly in the Global South, has to face the Eurocentric bias that universalizes Western notions of disability. This includes acknowledging the colonial medical narratives that created categories and justified interventions, which were disabling and devastating for the populations inhabiting the Global South (Grech, 2017; Meekosha, 2011; Roy, 2024).Indigenous disability activism in Latin America: Disability activists in Latin America, especially in Chile, have been actively involved in reivindicative occupational practices, struggling for acknowledgment and political power (Pino-Morán et al., 2023; Rebolledo-Sanhueza & Galaz-Valderrama, 2024). Indigenous disability militancy underscores intersectionality and decolonizing methods, making sure that research and policy are informed and guided by the ones who have gone through this experience (Daniels-Mayes, 2023). The attributes of resistance movement that took place in Latin America are depicted in Fig. 1.1.

Rights-based frameworks based on ancestral knowledge: The decolonization of disability through feminist thought in the Latin American context highlights new analytical categories that acknowledge the interrelation of colonialism, disability, and systemic inequalities (Ferrari, 2020). Rights-based approaches for disabled people must be based on the ancient wisdom and holistic view of well-being, holding legal provisions that sometimes are in contradiction with the definitions of disability in the social protection systems so far (Pinilla-Roncancio, 2015). Table 1.1 depicts the Indigenous Disability Activism in Latin America—Actors, Practices, and Decolonial Contributions.

Colonial medicine's contemporary legacies: The power of colonial medicine is still felt, albeit in various forms today, by which it is still making human life very hard for disabled persons in Latin America and keeping the latter groups in a very disadvantaged position (Lapierre, 2023).

Inequities among the health systems and the structural injustices: One of the significant issues faced by the health systems in Latin America is the fragmentation, which in turn results in quality gaps and sociopolitical-related upheaval, thus creating an enormous healthcare quartile (Roberti et al., 2024). Disabled individuals in Latin America and Caribbean countries very often are in the queue of the last ones to get healthcare access, and a shorter lifespan is the price they pay (Gatta et al., 2024; Reichenberger et al., 2024). It is quite evident that the above-mentioned structural inequities have their roots in the past and are a result of the continual dominance of colonial mentality, which is the prime element in the organizational setup of power, resources, and knowledge (Lapierre, 2023).

Environmental racism and the ongoing disablement: Latin America, to a great extent, is still plagued by the problem of environmental racism, which refers to the fact that certain groups of people are affected more than others by bad environmental situations and their disabling effects (Rougeon et al., 2023; Meireles et al., 2018).

Disability as a site of resistance where both politics and culture intertwine in the modern world: It's true that these difficulties have been around, but still, resistance in the form of political and cultural provocation is happening through disabilities. The situation and the power relations between the activists and authorities in Latin America are not only about the rights of disabled people but also the ongoing ones they are even fighting for the rights of the oppressed and the existing power structures (Pino-Morán et al., 2023; Rebolledo-Sanhueza & Galaz-Valderrama, 2024). One aspect of the Decolonial discourses is that it stirs the existing society and its analysis

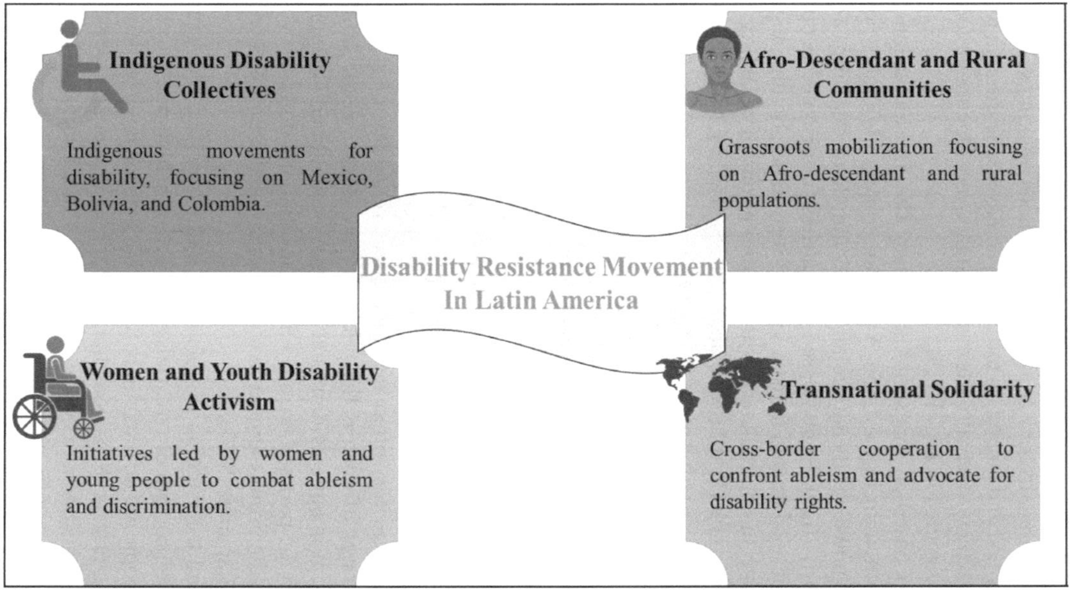

Fig. 1.1 Disability resistance movements in Latin America. The figure illustrates the diverse and intersecting strands of disability resistance movements across Latin America. This figure presents a conceptual map of disability resistance movements in Latin America, highlighting multiple, interconnected forms of activism. Indigenous Disability Collectives represent Indigenous-led movements addressing disability within cultural and territorial contexts, particularly in Mexico, Bolivia, and Colombia. Afro-descendant and Rural Communities emphasize grassroots mobilization focused on the lived experiences of Afro-descendant and rural populations. Women and Youth Disability Activism showcase initiatives led by women and young people aimed at challenging ableism and systemic discrimination. Transnational Solidarity reflects cross-border cooperation and alliances that confront ableism and advocate for disability rights at regional and global levels. The Disability Resistance Movement in Latin America signifies the convergence of these efforts into a broader, intersectional struggle for social justice, inclusion, and human rights for persons with disabilities

by insisting on the recognition that the knowledge produced by the oppressed people and their experiences is also significant for the culture and its transformation (Pino-Moran et al., 2023). The awareness provided by the social model of disability is at the core of this resistance, which not only makes it easier for people to request changes in society but also makes it easier for them to look for individual "cures."

1.5 Conclusion

Colonial medicine is not merely a neutral historical episode but a foundational force that is still influencing the perception, governance, and living of the disabled in Latin America today. The medicalization of disability, the racialization of bodies, and the preference for productivity over dignity were not unintentional colonial effects but rather implemented tactics that altered care into control. The same strategies of colonial rule still linger today in the forms of detached health systems, discriminatory laws, and persistent stigma around people with disabilities, especially those belonging to Indigenous, Afro-descendant, and poor communities. Thus, decolonizing disability entails more than just policy reform or legal recognition; it requires an epistemic shift. The Indigenous worldviews of health, which highlight interconnectedness, equilibrium, and the community's involvement, are great alternatives to Western biomedical reductionism. It is only through the colonial violence, environmental injustice, gendered control, and economic exploitation that we can see disability as a social construct, and old deficit-centered frameworks give way to justice-centered approaches. Importantly, disabled people in Latin America are not just symbols of powerlessness but also areas of resistance. The caring by the community, the coexistence of different medical practices, the participation in political movements by feminists and indigenous people, and the use of rights-based fights that rest on the foundation of ancestral knowledge are all showcasing that alternative futures are already being practiced. We maintain that reclaiming these counter-epistemologies is not only essential for disability justice but also for the larger decolonial transformations that continue to confront the deep-rooted power, knowledge, and value hierarchies.

References

Acevedo, M. L., García, X. E., & Moctezuma, A. (2023). Violencias de género hacia mujeres y niñas indígenas con discapacidad en América Latina. *Cahiers Franco-Latino-Américains D'études Sur Le Handicap, 1*, 18. https://doi.org/10.56078/cfla_discapacidad.159

Angarita-Cañas, P. E. (2020). Forced displacement and globalization in Latin America. In *The Oxford handbook of the sociology of Latin America*. https://doi.org/10.1093/oxfordhb/9780190926557.001.0001

Ashmead, A. S. (1894). Leprosy in America before the advent of the spaniards and the negroes. *Journal of the American Medical Association, 23*(23), 847–849.

Ashmead, A. S. (1895). Pre-columbian leprosy. *Journal of the American Medical Association, 24*(21), 803–807.

Bachfischer, A., Barbosa, M. C., Rojas, A. A. R., Bechler, R., Schwienhorst-Stich, E. M., Kasang, C., et al. (2023). Implementing community based inclusive development for people with disability in Latin America: A mixed methods perspective on prioritized needs and lessons learned. *International Journal for Equity in Health, 22*(1), 147. https://doi.org/10.1186/s12939-023-01966-8

Baez, M. L. B., Ramos, S. M., & del Valle Vasquez, E. (2024). Traditional medicine in Latin America: A holistic approach to health. *Community and Interculturality in Dialogue, 4*, 120–120. https://doi.org/10.56294/cid2024120

Barclay, J. L. (2017). Differently abled: Africanisms, disability, and power in the age of transatlantic slavery. In *Bioarchaeology of impairment and disability: Theoretical, ethnohistorical, and methodological perspectives* (pp. 77–94). Springer International Publishing. https://doi.org/10.1007/978-3-319-56949-9_5

Bautista-Valarezo, E., Duque, V., Verhoeven, V., Mejia Chicaiza, J., Hendrickx, K., Maldonado-Rengel, R., & Michels, N. R. (2021). Perceptions of ecuadorian indigenous healers on their relationship with the formal health care system: Barriers and opportunities. *BMC Complementary Medicine and Therapies, 21*(1), 65. https://doi.org/10.1186/s12906-021-03234-0

Block, P. (2007). Institutional utopias, eugenics, and intellectual disability in Brazil. *History and Anthropology, 18*(2), 177–196. https://doi.org/10.1080/02757200701702851

Boodman, E. (2023). Medical colonialism and the power to care: Unsettling participatory inclusion in the settler-state care paradigm. *Hypatia, 38*(2), 330–352. https://doi.org/10.1017/hyp.2023.24

Boveda, M., Reyes, G., & Aronson, B. (2019). Disciplined to access the general education curriculum: Girls of color, disabilities, and specialized education programming. *Curriculum Inquiry, 49*(4), 405–425. https://doi.org/10.1080/03626784.2019.1652543

Brégain, G., Venturiello, M. P., Ferrante, C., & Fuente-Alba, L. V. (2022). Les actions protestataires des personnes handicapées en Bolivie, au Chili et en Argentine. *Canadian Journal of Latin American and Caribbean Studies/Revue canadienne des études latino-américaines et caraïbes, 47*(3), 369–389. https://doi.org/10.1080/08263663.2022.2110746

Brieger, G. H. (2004). Bodies and borders: A new cultural history of medicine. *Perspectives in Biology and Medicine, 47*(3), 402–421. https://doi.org/10.1353/pbm.2004.0044

Brueggemann, A. D., & Ekwonye, A. U. (2023, December). Perceived benefits of magdalena energy healing sessions: An exploratory study of clients' perspectives. In *Healthcare* (Vol. 11, No. 23, p. 3087). doi:https://doi.org/10.3390/healthcare11233087.

Bueno, X., & Pardo, I. (2023). Gender-role attitudes and fertility ideals in Latin America. *Journal of Population Research, 40*(1), 2. https://doi.org/10.1007/s12546-023-09295-x

Carey, D., Jr. (2019). The politics and culture of medicine and disease in Central America. In *Oxford research encyclopedia of Latin American history*. https://doi.org/10.1093/acrefore/9780199366439.013.52

Chan, J., Griffiths, K., Turner, A., Tobias, J., Clarmont, W., Delaney, G., et al. (2023). Radiation therapy and indigenous peoples in Canada and Australia: Building paths toward reconciliation in cancer care delivery. *International Journal of Radiation Oncology* Biology* Physics, 116*(2), 421–429. https://doi.org/10.1016/j.ijrobp.2022.09.085

Chandanabhumma, P. P., & Narasimhan, S. (2020). Towards health equity and social justice: An applied framework of decolonization in health promotion. *Health Promotion International, 35*(4), 831–840. https://doi.org/10.1093/heapro/daz053

Chaves, M. (2022). Discapacidades y ciencias sociales. Interpelaciones en clave latinoamericana: Sobre discapacidades, prácticas e investigación: Interpelando a las ciencias sociales, de Andrea Verónica Pérez y Antonella Rapanelli (Compiladoras.). Santiago de chile: Ediciones CELEI y Centro de Estudios Latinoamericanos de Educación Inclusiva (CELEI), 2021. *Educación y vínculos. Revista de estudios interdisciplinarios en educación* (pp. 121–127). https://doi.org/10.33255/2591/1295

Connell, R. (2011). Southern bodies and disability: Re-thinking concepts. *Third World Quarterly, 32*(8), 1369–1381. https://doi.org/10.1080/01436597.2011.614799

Crocetti, A. C., Walker, T., Mitchell, F., Sherriff, S., Hill, K., Paradies, Y., et al. (2024). Making big business everybody's business: Aboriginal leaders' perspectives on commercial activities influencing aboriginal health in Victoria, Australia. *Globalization and Health, 20*(1), 33. https://doi.org/10.1186/s12992-024-01038-8

Dale, G. (2014). The iron law of democratic socialism: British and Austrian influences on the young Karl Polanyi. *Economy and Society, 43*(4), 650–667. https://doi.org/10.1080/03085147.2014.898821

Daniels-Mayes, S. (2023). Researching indigenous people living with a disability: The urgent need for an intersectional and decolonising approach (BlakAbility). *First Nations Health and Wellbeing-The Lowitja Journal, 1*, 100004. https://doi.org/10.1016/j.fnhli.2023.100004

de Freitas, M. H., Vilela, P. R., & Nwora, E. I. (2023). Religiosity and indigenous cosmology in a Brazilian hospital setting: The challenges faced by health professionals. *International Journal of Latin American Religions, 7*(1), 46–77. https://doi.org/10.1007/s41603-023-00194-w

de Souza, D. C. I., Vieira, V., & Hoepers, I. D. S. (2021). Afrodescendentes na América Latina: da liberdade aos processos de (in) exclusão. *Dialogia, 38*, e20455–e20455. https://doi.org/10.5585/38.2021.20455

Devakumar, D., Selvarajah, S., Abubakar, I., Kim, S. S., McKee, M., Sabharwal, N. S., et al. (2022). Racism, xenophobia, discrimination, and the determination of health. *The Lancet, 400*(10368), 2097–2108. https://doi.org/10.1016/S0140-6736(22)01972-9

Dirth, T. P., & Adams, G. A. (2019). Decolonial theory and disability studies: On the modernity/coloniality of ability. *Journal of Social and Political Psychology, 7*(1), 260–289. https://doi.org/10.5964/jspp.v7i1.762

Ferrari, M. B. (2020). Feminismos descoloniales y discapacidad: hacia una conceptualización de la colonialidad de la capacidad. *Nómadas, 52*, 115–131. https://doi.org/10.30578/nomadas.n52a7

Franceschet, S., & Thomas, G. (2016). Gender, politics, and the state in Latin America. *The Wiley Blackwell Encyclopedia of Gender and Sexuality Studies*, 1–9. https://doi.org/10.1002/9781118663219.wbegss581

Fredrick, S. (2021). Mayan and Andean medicine and urban space in the Spanish Americas. *Renaissance and reformation, 44*(2), 147–181. https://doi.org/10.33137/rr.v44i2.37524

Gatta, D. R., Rotenberg, S., Allel, K., Reichenberger, V., Banks, L. M., & Kuper, H. (2024). Access to general health care among people with disabilities in Latin America and the Caribbean: A systematic review of quantitative research. *The Lancet Regional Health–Americas*, 32. https://doi.org/10.1016/j.lana.2024.100701

Goikolea-Amiano, I. (2020). Decolonising through historicising. *AYER, 117*, 351–365. http://revistaayer.com/articulo/1407

González-Calle, J. L., Sánchez Contreras, C. A., & Monteserín Abella, O. (2023). The nature and production of urban space in Latin America: A historical review of the case of Ibagué (Colombia). *Land, 12*(9), 1807. https://doi.org/10.3390/land12091807

Grech, S. (2017). Decolonising eurocentric disability studies: Why colonialism matters in the disability and global south debate. In *Disability and colonialism* (pp. 6–21). Routledge. https://doi.org/10.1080/13504630.2014.995347

Grieshaber, E. P. (1979). Hacienda—Indian community relations and Indian acculturation: An historiographical essay. *Latin American Research Review, 14*(3), 107–128. https://www.cist-regards.fr/opac_css/index.php?lvl=bulletin_display&id=11006

Harding, S. (2016). Latin American decolonial social studies of scientific knowledge: Alliances and tensions. *Science, Technology, & Human Values, 41*(6), 1063–1087. https://doi.org/10.1177/0162243916656465

Hernández, F. A., Chamorro, J. M., & Pastas, N. M. (2024). Spiritual disharmonies among the emberá dobida: Territorial, bodily, and linguistic suffering. *Journal of Applied Youth Studies, 7*(1), 27–46. https://doi.org/10.1007/s43151-023-00111-0

Hutcheon, E. J., & Lashewicz, B. (2020). Tracing and troubling continuities between ableism and colonialism in Canada. *Disability & Society, 35*(5), 695–714. https://doi.org/10.1080/09687599.2019.1647145

Janka, C., Höcker, M., & Dorner, T. E. (2024). The relationship between body, mind, and social characteristics in a sample of a training program for developing social and personal resources: A network analysis. *International Journal of Environmental Research and Public Health, 21*(12), 1654. https://doi.org/10.3390/ijerph21121654

Javier, S. J., Perrin, P. B., Snipes, D. J., Olivera, S. L., Perdomo, J. L., Arango, J. A., & Arango-Lasprilla, J. C. (2013). The influence of health related quality of life on sexual desire in individuals with spinal cord injury from Colombia, South America. *Sexuality and Disability, 31*(4), 325–335. https://doi.org/10.1007/s11195-013-9320-x

Kerr, A. E. (2020). Trust Me, I'ma Doctor. *Latin American Literary Review, 47*(93), 2–11.

Lapierre, M. (2023). Disability and Latin American indigenous peoples. *Disability & Society, 38*(7), 1276–1280. https://doi.org/10.1080/09687599.2023.2192381

Lara, I. (2008). Latina health activist-healers bridging body and spirit. *Women & Therapy, 31*(1), 21–40. https://doi.org/10.1300/02703140802145169

Linett, M. T. (2024). Disability untheorized: Critiques of eugenics, then and now. *CUSP: Late Nineteenth and Early Twentieth Century Cultures, 2*(2), 172–183.

Lovern, L. L. (2017). Indigenous perspectives on difference: A case for inclusion. *Journal of Literary & Cultural Disability Studies, 11*(3), 303–320. https://doi.org/10.3828/jlcds.2017.24

Lovern, L. L. (2022). Indigenous concepts of difference: An alternative to Western disability labeling. *Disability Studies Quarterly, 41*(4). https://doi.org/10.18061/dsq.v41i4.8468

Meekosha, H. (2011). Decolonising disability: Thinking and acting globally. *Disability & Society, 26*(6), 667–682. https://doi.org/10.1080/09687599.2011.602860

Meireles, A. J. D. A., Melo, J. A. T., & Said, M. A. (2018). Environmental injustice in Northeast Brazil: The Pecém industrial and shipping complex. In *Environmental impacts of transnational corporations in the global south* (pp. 171–187). Emerald Publishing Limited. https://doi.org/10.1108/S0161-723020180000033007

Menéndez, E. L. (2015). Las enfermedades¿ son solo padecimientos?: biomedicina, formas de atención" paralelas" y proyectos de poder. *Salud colectiva, 11*, 301–330. https://doi.org/10.18294/sc.2015.719

Mercadante, M. T., Evans-Lacko, S., & Paula, C. S. (2009). Perspectives of intellectual disability in Latin American countries: Epidemiology, policy, and services for children and adults. *Current Opinion in Psychiatry, 22*(5), 469–474. https://doi.org/10.1097/YCO.0b013e32832eb8c6

Mignolo, W. (2000). *Border thinking and the colonial difference* (pp. 49–90). Local Histories/Global Desings: Coloniality, Subaltern Knowledges and Border Thinking.

Musante, K. (2019). Indigenous peoples, postcolonial ontologies, neoliberal regimes, and approaches to understanding medical pluralism in Latin America. *Latin American Research Review, 54*(1), 269–276. https://doi.org/10.25222/larr.790

Newson, L. A. (2006). Medical practice in early colonial Spanish America: A prospectus. *Bulletin of Latin American Research, 25*(3), 367–391. https://doi.org/10.1111/j.0261-3050.2006.00203.x

Ortega, D. C. V. (2023). Tierra de imbunches y ch'uqtas: la dis-capacidad como dispositivo colonial en América Latina y el Caribe. *Brazilian Journal of Latin American Studies, 22*(47), 197–222. https://doi.org/10.11606/issn.1676-6288.prolam.23.213227

Papalini, V., & Avelín Cesco, M. J. (2022). Pluralismo médico: regulaciones y concepciones de salud en seis países de América Latina. *Perfiles Latinoamericanos, 30*(59). https://doi.org/10.18504/pl3059-009-2022

Pinilla-Roncancio, M. (2015). Disability and social protection in Latin American countries. *Disability & Society, 30*(7), 1005–1020. https://doi.org/10.1080/09687599.2015.1059316

Pino-Moran, J. A., Rodriguez-Garrido, P., & Lapierre, M. (2023). Wild, indigenous, lame, invalid: Anti-ableist epistemologies of the south. *Saúde e Sociedade, 32*, e211010es. https://doi.org/10.1590/S0104-12902023211010en

Pino-Morán, J. A., Zango-Martin, I., Rodríguez-Garrido, P., & Mora-Malo, E. (2023). Reivindicative occupational practices of activist with disabilities. *Cadernos Brasileiros de Terapia Ocupacional, 31*, e3510. https://doi.org/10.1590/2526-8910.ctoAO269135102

Plaisime, M. V., Jipguep-Akhtar, M. C., & Belcher, H. M. (2023). 'White people are the default': A qualitative analysis of medical trainees' perceptions of cultural competency, medical culture, and racial bias. *SSM-Qualitative Research in Health, 4*, 100312. https://doi.org/10.1016/j.ssmqr.2023.100312

Puszka, S., Walsh, C., Markham, F., Barney, J., Yap, M., & Dreise, T. (2022). Towards the decolonisation of disability: A systematic review of disability conceptualisations, practices and experiences of first nations people of Australia. *Social Science & Medicine, 305*, 115047. https://doi.org/10.1016/j.socscimed.2022.115047

Ramos, C. (2021). Beyond the Columbian exchange: Medicine and public health in colonial Latin America. *History compass, 19*(8), e12682. https://doi.org/10.1111/hic3.12682

Rebolledo-Sanhueza, J. A., & Galaz-Valderrama, C. (2024). Activismo y discapacidad en Latinoamérica: luchas por el reconocimiento. *Revista Estudos Feministas, 32*(1). https://doi.org/10.1590/1806-9584-2024v32n190769

Reichenberger, V., Corona, A. P., Ramos, V. D., Shakespeare, T., Hameed, S., Penn-Kekana, L., & Kuper, H. (2024). Access to primary healthcare services for adults with disabilities in Latin America and the Caribbean: A review and meta-synthesis of qualitative studies. *Disability and Rehabilitation, 46*(25), 6011–6020. https://doi.org/10.1080/09638288.2024.2320268

Roberti, J., Leslie, H. H., Doubova, S. V., Ranilla, J. M., Mazzoni, A., Espinoza, L., et al. (2024). Inequalities in health system coverage and quality: A cross-sectional survey of four Latin American countries. *The Lancet Global Health, 12*(1), e145–e155. https://doi.org/10.1016/S2214-109X(23)00488-6

Rodríguez, L. C. (2020). Inappropriate/d bodies: Reorganizing the terms of life and death. *Death Studies, 44*(11), 727–735. https://doi.org/10.1080/07481187.2020.1771854

Rosales-Rivadeneira, S., Álvarez-Moreno, M., & Tito-Pineda, P. (2017). Indigenous cosmovision about health and illness in Otavalo-Ecuador. *Procedia-Social and Behavioral Sciences, 237*, 975–979. https://doi.org/10.1016/j.sbspro.2017.02.138

Rougeon, M., Mota, C., & Trad, L. (2023). Environmental racism and environmental justice: Decolonial inflections and new agendas in Latin America and Brazil. *Journal of Political Ecology, 30*(1), 699–715. https://doi.org/10.2458/jpe.5863

Roy, A. (2024). Decolonizing disability studies: Identities, epistemologies and global south perspectives. *The Creative Launcher, 9*(6), 70–81. https://doi.org/10.53032/tcl.2024.9.6.07

Sanmiquel-Molinero, L., Pujol-Tarrés, J., & Montenegro, M. (2023). Latin American perspectives on parenthood and disability: Vulnerability, risk, and social inclusion. *Social Inclusion, 11*(4), 338–349. https://doi.org/10.17645/si.v11i4.7046

Schiappacasse, C., Guzmán, J. M., Dean, M. H., Corletto, S., Battistella, L. R., Imamura, M., et al. (2019). Physical medicine and rehabilitation in Latin America: Development and current status. *Physical Medicine and Rehabilitation Clinics of North America, 30*(4), 749–755. https://doi.org/10.1016/j.pmr.2019.07.001

Schleck, G., & Ben-Alon, L. (2024). Eco-ableism and access circularity in natural building. *Frontiers of Architectural Research, 13*(2), 235–248. https://doi.org/10.1016/j.foar.2023.11.005

Schmidt, B. E. (2021). Spiritual healing in Latin America. In *The Routledge handbook of religion, medicine, and health* (pp. 113–125). Routledge. https://doi.org/10.4324/9781315207964

Seaton, A. (2020). The gospel of wealth and the national health: The Rockefeller foundation and social medicine in Britain's NHS, 1945–60. *Bulletin of the History of Medicine, 94*(1), 91–124. https://doi.org/10.1353/bhm.2020.0003

Senier, S. (2013). "Traditionally, disability was not seen as such" writing and healing in the work of Mohegan medicine people. *Journal of Literary & Cultural Disability Studies, 7*(2), 213–229. https://doi.org/10.3828/jlcds.2013.15

Sepúlveda Jara, R., & Oyarce Pisani, A. M. (2020). New and old knowledge aimed at decolonising mental health: Reflections and proposals from Chile. *International Review of Psychiatry, 32*(4), 334–339. https://doi.org/10.1080/09540261.2020.1767042

Setio, R. (2026). Decolonizing disability in social and theology structures: An Indonesian Perspective1. *Journal of Disability & Religion, 30*(1), 81–99. https://doi.org/10.1080/23312521.2025.2531798

Solsona-Cisternas, D. A. (2025). Individuation processes in disabled people. An approach through mobilities in rural areas of southern Chile. *Disability & Society, 40*(1), 47–69. https://doi.org/10.1080/09687599.2023.2263632

Sowell, D. (2003). Contending medical ideologies and state formation: The nineteenth-century origins of medical pluralism in contemporary Colombia. *Bulletin of the History of Medicine, 77*(4), 900–926. https://doi.org/10.1353/bhm.2003.0194

Stern, A. M. (2016). Eugenics in Latin America. In *Oxford Research Encyclopedia of Latin American History*. https://doi.org/10.1093/acrefore/9780199366439.013.315

Stienstra, D., & Ashcroft, T. (2010). Voyaging on the seas of spirit: An ongoing journey towards understanding disability and humanity. *Disability & Society, 25*(2), 191–203. https://doi.org/10.1080/09687590903534411

Summerhill, W. R. (1800). Railroads in imperial Brazil, 1854–1889. *Latin America and the World Economy Since*, 389–405.

Sundberg, J. (2008). Placing race in environmental justice research in Latin America. *Society and Natural Resources, 21*(7), 569–582. https://doi.org/10.1080/08941920802111538

Velarde, M. R. (2018). Indigenous perspectives of disability. *Disability Studies Quarterly, 38*(4). https://doi.org/10.18061/dsq.v38i4.6114

Vrana, H. (2023). Endemic goiter and El Salvador's battle against cretinismo. *The American Historical Review, 128*(4), 1587–1617. https://doi.org/10.1093/ahr/rhad377

Walin, M. (2023). Who should procreate? Selecting the best breeders through the control of marriage, Spain 1850s–1920s. *Journal of Iberian and Latin American Studies, 29*(1), 91–113. https://doi.org/10.1080/14701847.2023.2184018

Walsh, S. (2019a). Restoring the Chilean race: Catholicism and Latin eugenics in Chile. *The Catholic Historical Review*, 116–138. https://doi.org/10.1353/cat.2019.0047

Walsh, S. (2019b). The Chilean exception: Racial homogeneity, mestizaje and eugenic nationalism. *Journal of Iberian and Latin American Studies, 25*(1), 105–125. https://doi.org/10.1080/14701847.2019.1579499

Weaver, H. N. (2015). Disability through a native American lens: Examining influences of culture and colonization. *Journal of Social Work in Disability & Rehabilitation, 14*(3–4), 148–162. https://doi.org/10.1080/1536710X.2015.1068256

Woods, R., Milton, D., Arnold, L., & Graby, S. (2018). Redefining critical autism studies: A more inclusive interpretation. *Disability & Society, 33*(6), 974–979. https://doi.org/10.1080/09687599.2018.1454380

Yarza de los Ríos, A. (2020). Aɨdaɨza y baa wa waljai wa wa: relatos, visiones y entramados sobre" discapacidad" desde dos mundos indígenas en Colombia. *Nómadas, 52*, 81–95. https://doi.org/10.30578/nomadas.n52a5

Zaks, Z. (2024). Changing the medical model of disability to the normalization model of disability: Clarifying the past to create a new future direction. *Disability & Society, 39*(12), 3233–3260. https://doi.org/10.1080/09687599.2023.2255926

Chapter 2
Disability, Race, and Class: Intersections of Oppression in Latin America

Abstract In this chapter, disability is considered the main intersection of different forms of oppression in Latin America, situated right at the crossroads of race, class, and coloniality. This whole argument is rooted in the concepts of intersectionality, decoloniality, and critiques from Latin America; the chapter not only poses a challenge against the biomedical and individualizing models of disability but also points out the temporal and structural factors that facilitate its existence in racially defined capitalism, in extractive industries, and among the power relations of the colonial past that are still in place. It discusses how differently disability has been associated with race by colonial mechanisms that determine which bodies should be regarded as productive, usual, and human, and how these mechanisms persist through labor exploitation, environmental racism, poverty, informality, and the inability to access healthcare, education, and legal systems. The chapter asserts that the Indigenous and Afro-descendant communities are the hardest hit by the disability limitations, as they are always the first to suffer the consequences of land grabbing, residing in contaminated areas, working in low-paid jobs, and being denied the right to speak and have their knowledge acknowledged. It also highlights the movement of collective struggles, community-based caring, and decolonial practices that change the perception of disability from a liability to a source of knowledge, unity, and political power. By framing disability justice within the broader context of struggles against racial, economic, and epistemological oppression, the chapter presents a radical new view of social justice in Latin America through decolonial and intersectional lenses.

Keywords Disability · Intersectionality · Coloniality · Disability justice · Latin America

2.1 Introduction

The whole idea of intersectionality shines a spotlight on the fact that inequality dynamics can't be divided into separate categories but exist side by side. During the late 1980s and early 1990s, the term "intersectionality" gained popularity thanks

S. M. Thomas and R. Veerabathiran, *Disability and Decolonial Thought in Latin America*, SpringerBriefs in Modern Perspectives on Disability Research,
https://doi.org/10.1007/978-981-95-8950-0_2

to a legal scholar, Kimberlé Crenshaw, who wanted to bring an issue that was so prevalent among black women in the U.S., but which was almost invisibly present, to a larger audience through her analytical framework, focusing on the injustices stemming from race and gender. Alongside Crenshaw, intersectional theorists such as Collins (2000) and Choo and Ferree (2010) have reformulated their ideas about the universalization of racial and gendered subjects in feminist and critical race research; they have proposed a more nuanced representation, in which white women stand for only one part of all the women and black men only for one part of all the blacks. The models of disability are depicted in Fig. 2.1.

Thus, intersectionality has not only become a significant subject of research and theory but also led researchers to apply intersectional lenses to an increasingly broader range of processes and identities. However, disability still seems to be a blind spot in the intersectionality debate, more so in the field of sociology, the reason probably being that sociology has hardly considered disability as a separate social inequality category at all. Intersecting race and disability remain a relatively under-explored area in sociological studies. Gender and disability have been very rarely studied together, though, and when so, their connection has not usually been analyzed through the lens of an intersectional race and disability approach but instead restricted to health-related issues. This is surprising since, in the sociological field, racism and ableism interact strongly and are thus involved in many topics of great concern, such as mass incarceration and the school-to-prison pipeline (Frederick, 2017; Frederick & Shifrer, 2019; Gerschick & Stevens, 2016; Hammer, 2012; Maroto & Pettinicchio, 2015; Phelan et al., 2008).

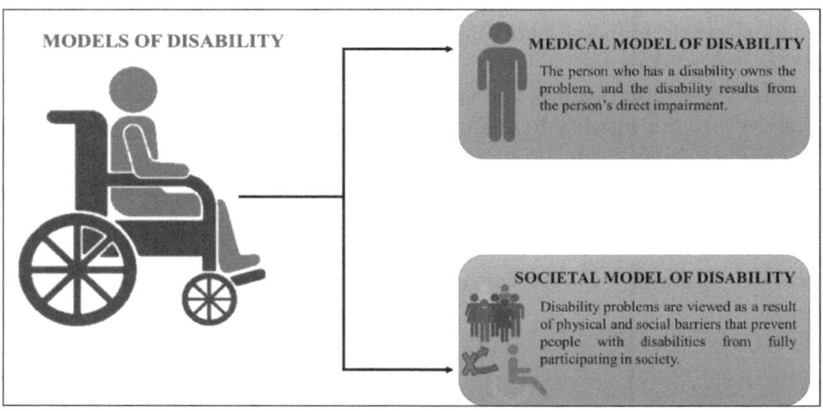

Fig. 2.1 Models of disability. The figure illustrates two contrasting frameworks used to understand disability: the Medical Model and the Societal (Social) Model. The Medical Model of Disability conceptualizes disability as a problem located within the individual, arising directly from a physical, sensory, or cognitive impairment, and emphasizes diagnosis, treatment, or cure. In contrast, the Societal Model of Disability views disability as the result of social, environmental, and physical barriers that restrict the participation of individuals with impairments in society

Decolonial scholarship has placed ever greater emphasis on the point that disability can neither be considered nor discussed as a neutral and purely biomedical condition and has to be placed within the still-existing structures of coloniality that organize race, class, gender, and even knowledge itself. To Reed-Sandoval and Sirvent, disability is not only influenced by racialized, gendered, and sexual hierarchies, but it is also, as a result of the coloniality of power, that defines whose bodies are normal, productive, and human—that is, the power of the coloniality of power. According to the authors, the idea of mestiza consciousness put forth by Gloria Anzaldúa is an excellent metaphor for how disabled, racialized, and working-class bodies can be seen as occupying the "underside of modernity," where being excluded from the dominant ways of thinking and knowing becomes a place of embodied knowledge, resistance, and alliance at the same time. The current view has also taken hold in Latin America, where racialized capitalism, extractive economies, and Eurocentric legal and medical systems are still among the factors that push Indigenous and Afro-descendant disabled bodies to be treated as non-existent, dispensable, or morbid. This chapter acknowledges and analyzes coloniality as a structure that is at once epistemic, political, and economic, and hence approaches disability as the intersection of race, class, and historical domination rather than as an individual deficit, thus locating the issue of disability justice squarely within the larger fight for decolonial social transformation (Reed-Sandoval & Sirvent, 2019).

This chapter aims to cast the disability issue in a new light, highlighting it as the main—rather than secondary—axis of intersectional oppression in Latin America. Most importantly, it still leads the discourse, bearing in mind the socio-theoretical and historical perspectives. It would demonstrate how disability is not only lived but also governed in the dualistic perspective of race, class, and colonialism in the given context of racial capitalism, extractive economies, and socially exclusionary practices. The theoretical discussion would be informed by decolonization theory, intersectionality, and Latin American critical scholarship, which not only portray disability as a social and historical phenomenon but also claim its rightful place in the discourse on justice and rights through the lens of disability justice. The chapter has no intention of becoming a mere debater of biomedical and individualizing views regarding disability. However, it will involve broader debates around disability justice, highlight modes of resistance and people's power, and contribute to the picture of social justice from a perspective that is both decolonial and recognizes disability as intertwined with the struggles against inequality and the erasure of the oppressed in Latin America.

2.2 Racialization of Disability and Colonial Legacies

The racialization of disability in Latin America is a phenomenon that has its roots deeply entrenched in the historical and present-day colonial domination tactics that heavily rely on race, gender, class, and bodily ability to organize society's hierarchy. Aníbal Quijano's idea of coloniality posits that such domination takes place through the establishment of classifications and hierarchies that assign different levels of humanity and worth to various groups of people. In this perspective, race became the leading factor through which colonialism set up labor, knowledge, and social connections, thereby justifying the taking over and oppression of the indigenous population (Quijano, 2000, 2005). This same discrimination against people with disabilities is based on the same reasoning, not as an impartial medical condition, but as a socially created stigma of inferiority linked with the oppression of the racialized group.

Modernity in the colonial context was built upon the notion that the European, white, male, and capable individuals were the standard of humanity. All the other human forms—Indigenous, Black, colonized, women, or poor people—were, however, represented as lacking, irrational, and incapacitated to different extents. In the works of Mignolo (2009, 2017), one can find the argument that coloniality represents the "dark side" of modernity, and that it is the latter that produces various forms of knowledge that keep oppressors in control while making subaltern bodies and their ways of knowing invisible. Disability can be seen as one of the main factors that not only made racialized communities a subject of medical concern but also their consequent exclusion from taking part in all aspects of society and politics.

The historical narrations of colonial encounters in Latin America showcase the fact that racialized bodies were very often classified through the concepts of monstrosity, degeneration, and abnormality. The author Lilia Lobo, in her analysis of travelers' narratives, refers to people belonging to the Indigenous tribes, enslaved Africans, poor people, and those who were referred to as "idiots" or "mad" as being depicted as living at the borderline of human and animal. Such representations were not mere metaphors; they were rooted in European scientific and philosophical discourses that characterized physical and mental differences as signs of racial inferiority (Gesser et al., 2024; Silva, 2011). Therefore, disability played the role of a racializing technology, which, through the merging of non-whiteness and incapacity, further strengthened colonial hierarchies.

In the viewpoints of decolonial feminist scholars, coloniality generates individuals who are at the same time racialized, sexualized, impoverished, and dehumanized. Curiel (2020) underscores how colonial power metamorphoses certain groups into objects of knowledge, intervention, and control rather than acknowledging them as political and epistemic agents. Disability in this scenario is used to rationalize exclusion and violence against those who are considered to be not only an associative hindrance to modernization but also a drain on capital productivity. The whole process takes place in a way that, through the positioning of the racialized populations, they not only lose their productive capacities but also become a burden on the social strata, thus further strengthening the race-disability association in the colonial imaginary.

The idea of coloniality of ability, proposed by Ferrari (2020), offers a fresh perspective on how the birth of disability was linked to the colonial rule of the earth. In her case, Ferrari says that colonial modernity not only toppled pre-colonial communal ethics of reciprocity, cooperation, and collective responsibility but also, the very demise of such ethics changed the whole racial hierarchy, as Indigenous and Afro-descendant people lost their social organization patterns and were put under the regimes that considered human beings worthless if they could not or did not want to keep up with the capitalist norms of labor. Therefore, the power of the colonial relations was such that disability became a structural production rather than a mere imposition on individual bodies.

The disability racialization process is furthered through the coloniality of knowledge. Grosfoguel (2016) states that the basic assumption of Western epistemologies is that they come from genocide and epistemicide that keep the knowledge of white European males at the top while disqualifying others' ways of knowing. This hierarchy of knowledge permits the use of scientific racism, medicalization, and normalization practices that depict racialized and disabled bodies as pathological deviations. The use of these techniques can be traced back to the period of psychiatric institutionalization in Latin America, where it was mainly Black, Indigenous, poor, and socially non-conforming people who were imprisoned in asylums under the pretext of treatment (Arbex, 2019). Such institutions were places of social cleansing, reinforcing the idea that some lives were not worth protecting or caring for.

It is important to note that the pre-colonial Latin American societies did not always view bodily differences as shortcomings. Ferrari (2020) notes that in certain Indigenous worldviews, unusual physical traits may be seen as indicators of a person's spiritual superiority or their importance in the community. The colonial rule forced upon Europeans the biomedical and moral frameworks that completely wiped out these other ways of seeing, thus establishing a single model of ability based on racialized ideas of progress and civilization. This breaking of knowledge points to the colonial roots of modern-day ableism and its linkage with race and class oppression.

The listing of disability as a colonial and racialized category gives rise to a new interpretation of the Eurocentric disability paradigms and promotes an intersectional, decolonial approach based on Latin American realities. The authors, Collins and Bilge (2021), assert that intersectionality should reflect the mutual construction of power systems rather than an additive approach to social categories. In the case of Latin America, the issue of disability is inseparable from the historical background of racial violence, economic exploitation, and epistemic exclusion. So, the disability justice conversation has to deal with the colonial legacies that still determine who gets to be considered capable, human, and socially belonging.

The racialization of disability in Latin America is one of the cornerstones of modern/colonial capitalism. Disability, race, and class are interrelated factors through which oppression operates, producing a hierarchy of humanity and justifying exclusion and violence. A decolonial perspective uncovers these mechanisms and enables thinking of disability not as a deficit or tragedy, but as a site of resilience, knowledge creation, and collective struggle.

2.3 Disability in Racialized Capitalism and Extractive Economies

In Latin America, disability under the racialized capitalism system is revealed as a means of subjugation, where the capitalist system not only intersects with race and class, but also the indigenous and Afro-descendant people are the ones who suffer the most through their exploitation and marginalization in resource extraction and labor. The economies of extraction intensify the disabling process by their operations in dangerous environments, and the significant impact of impairment is on racialized groups.

2.3.1 Extractivism, Land Dispossession, and Disabling Environments

In Latin America, the extractive industries are the main driving force behind large-scale resource extraction that eventually leads to land dispossession, thus destroying the native people's territories and making the surrounding areas physically unlivable. An example is the government of Ecuador's Yasuní-ITT region switching from oil preservation initiatives to prioritizing state finances after abandoning them, which, in turn, led to the disappearance of indigenous groups and the pollution of ecosystems vital to health and mobility. Neo-extractivism under progressive regimes, as in the case of Bolivia's TIPNIS highway project, continues to tap into the "remote" indigenous lands, causing loss of biodiversity and, at the same time, imposing chronic health impairments due to pollution and forced relocation. These developments lead to the establishment of "sacrifice zones," creating a situation where marginalized racialized communities are the first to suffer from disability and health-related issues because losing their lands cut them off from their traditional medicines and sustainable sources of income, thus, making ableism an inherent part of the colonial powers' hierarchies (Artiga-Purcell et al., 2023; Auz, 2024; Lapierre, 2023; Robeyns, 2025).

2.3.2 Labor Exploitation, Occupational Injury, and Class Vulnerability

The most severe kinds of labor exploitation are suffered by racialized workers in the mining and informal sectors of Latin America, leading to occupational injuries, which are the main cause of the disability of the same social class. Latino day laborers, who are mostly indigenous or mestizo, have the highest U.S. injury rates from working in unsafe construction without safety gear, which is the same pattern that can be found in Latin American scenarios like the industries along the Texas border. Intersectional capitalism directs the Latinx immigrants toward non-secure jobs such as construction and cleaning, where the citizen barrier obstructs the labor rights protection, leading to the workers' exhaustion and even chronic pain being categorized as a health condition. The basic workers during the pandemic were exposed to even higher risks; for example, the mining in Chile was linked to the spread of the virus and deaths, thus showing that class vulnerability of the workers racializes their injuries, which are a by-product of immigration policies (Artiga-Purcell et al., 2023; Fernández-Esquer et al., 2020; Iunes, 2002; Ruiz-Negrón et al., 2026). The comparative analysis of extractivism and labor exploitation is depicted in Table 2.1.

2.3.3 Environmental Racism, Toxicity, and Community Disablement

In Latin America, environmental racism is such a big issue that it has even been termed "racialized communities" to depict the situation, and toxics are the main agents behind it; thus, for example, people suffer as a whole through contaminated water and air. That is, for instance, in the case of the Indigenous peoples, they usually endure mercury, cyanide, and lead poisoning coming from mining, and the governments' decisions are pretty much in favor of the latter (i.e., mining) in the so-called "sacrifice zones." In places like urban basins with cities such as Buenos Aires and Bogotá, the less fortunate Afro-descendant and indigenous neighborhoods are living with untreated sewage and industrial waste all around them. Thus, amid health epidemics, they have to go to court and file lawsuits to protect their environmental rights. Also, the poor people living in these areas of agrochemicals and extractive spills suffer from respiratory diseases and disabilities, while the structural racism that is prevailing in the health care system really stops them from getting the treatment they need. All these toxicities reflect racial capitalism, in which the company's profits come at the expense of the health of marginalized communities (Auz, 2024; Beard et al., 2024; Féliz & Melón, 2023; Herrera, 2024; Rodríguez Aguilera, 2021; Telles et al., 2025).

2.4 Poverty, Informality, and the Political Economy of Disablement

Poverty and informality in Latin America are still the leading causes of disability by preventing social protections from being accessed by marginalized racial and class groups, thus keeping them in a state of vulnerability. Informal labor markets are the main ones, and they magnify the risk of disability, particularly for indigenous and Afro-descendants and the low-income workers, who are the most affected and least likely to have access to medical care or compensation for injuries. The burdens of

Table 2.1 Comparative analysis of extractivism and labor exploitation in the production of disability under racialized capitalism

Analytical dimension	Extractivism	Labor exploitation
Primary economic logic	Large-scale extraction of natural resources for global markets	Maximization of surplus value through precarious and unsafe labor
Main sites of operation	Indigenous territories, rural resource-rich regions, protected ecosystems	Mines, construction sites, agriculture, informal and cross-border labor markets
Key actors	Multinational corporations, state-owned extractive enterprises, national governments	Employers, subcontractors, informal labor brokers, state labor regulators
Targeted populations	Indigenous and afro-descendant communities living on or near extractive lands	Indigenous, mestizo, afro-descendant, migrant, and undocumented workers
Mechanism of racialization	Territories and bodies deemed "expendable" or "remote"	Workers racialized as disposable, cheap, and replaceable labor
Core form of dispossession	Loss of land, water, biodiversity, and territorial autonomy	Loss of labor rights, bodily integrity, and economic security
Typical disabling environments	Polluted soil and water, deforestation, toxic air, forced relocation	Unsafe workplaces, lack of protective equipment, excessive work hours
Forms of violence involved	Slow violence, environmental degradation, forced displacement	Direct bodily injury, exhaustion, repetitive strain, occupational accidents
Temporal nature of harm	Long-term and intergenerational	Immediate, cumulative, and chronic
Primary disability outcomes	Neurological damage, respiratory illness, mobility impairment, chronic disease	Musculoskeletal injury, chronic pain, trauma-related impairments
Relationship to environment	Disability produced through ecological destruction	Disability produced through bodily exploitation
Role of the state	Facilitates extraction through policy, militarization, and deregulation	Weak enforcement of labor protections; criminalization of migrants
Healthcare access	Severely limited due to remoteness and discrimination	Restricted by immigration status, informality, and class
Legal framing of harm	Often treated as "development trade-offs"	Framed as individual workplace accidents
Ableism produced	Communities labeled unproductive or backward once impaired	Workers blamed for injury or perceived lack of productivity

(continued)

Table 2.1 (continued)

Analytical dimension	Extractivism	Labor exploitation
Gendered dimensions	Women face reproductive harm and caregiving burdens	Men experience high injury rates; women concentrated in informal care and cleaning work
Pandemic intensification	Continued extraction despite public health risks	Essential workers exposed to heightened risk and mortality
Forms of resistance	Indigenous land defense, environmental justice movements	Labor organizing, migrant rights advocacy
Disability politics	Disability emerges as collective and territorial	Disability individualized and depoliticized
Outcome for capital accumulation	Profits externalized at the cost of community health	Profits generated through expendable labor bodies
Conceptual contribution to disability studies	Frames disability as environmental and territorial	Frames disability as occupational and class-based

care and the divides between urban and rural areas that are based on gender only serve to strengthen the inequalities, and along with race, to disable communities structurally (Duryea et al., 2019).

2.4.1 *Informal Labor Markets and Social Protection Exclusion*

Informal employment accounts for more than half of the workforce in Latin America, reaching 57–70% in countries like Bolivia and Honduras. Disabled workers in these countries are severely excluded from social security, pensions, and health insurance. People with disabilities in Latin America are around 85 million (14.7% of the population) and thus, most of them are in informal jobs—almost 68% of the working-age adults with disabilities are employed in such jobs—without contracts, safety nets, or any accommodations like the ones in formal employment. The political economy of disablement helps the racialized poor access only low-paid own-account work or family labor, where occupational hazards such as machinery accidents or chemical exposure are left uncompensated, which is already deep poverty and impairment (Pucheta & Kalil, 2025; Utzet et al., 2021).

Racial hierarchies make the situation worse for the minorities: Indigenous and Afro-Latinos, often working in urban services or rural agriculture, are often working in even more informal conditions with their rate going up to 70%, while the households that totally depend on such income have 45% of their members being children and elderly, making the situation even worse by heightening intergenerational disablement. In the absence of contributory schemes, disabilities resulting from untreated illnesses or injuries become permanent, as in mixed households where formal workers subsidize informal kin but cannot bridge the systemic gaps (Duryea et al., 2019; OECD, 2025).

2.4.2 Gendered Dimensions of Disability, Care, and Class Inequality

In Latin America, women with disabilities are, however, unfairly treated as they shoulder the most significant part of the care burden in informal economies, where not only the class issue but also the race issue magnifies the effects of unpaid reproductive labor through cycles of exhaustion and health decline. The gender pay gap is one of the factors that makes the impact of informality larger for women. Women with disabilities are twice as likely not to be employed or educated; thus, they are accustomed to low-wage domestic or street vending while taking care of their disabled relatives. For example, indigenous women in Peru or Guatemala do informal farming and at the same time take care of older people and children, thus, they are facing mobility problems caused by malnutrition or overwork without any support from the government at the same time (Bachfischer et al., 2023; Stlouka et al., 2024).

The class disparity is, however, evident as racialized women in informal households are the ones who absorb the care deficits, where 71% of informal workers live, limiting access to formal care services and creating more dependency. This gendered disablement is in tune with capitalist extraction, which considers women's bodies as non-productive and therefore, they are not entitled to formal protections that are biased toward urban, mestizo men (Duryea et al., 2019; Purfield, 2006).

2.4.3 Rural-Urban Disparities and Regional Inequalities

Latin America's rural landscape shows a stark contrast in disability, with 75–80% informality in Central America and Andean agricultural regions, while urban averages stand at 50–60%. Notably, Indigenous rural communities are a source of 25% informal agricultural labor, thus being the most susceptible to health issues due to pesticides and ergonomic strains. Still, they are deprived of proper treatment and forced into urban migration, which directs them to city slums where they can find unauthorized construction work without any kind of protection. Regional inequalities are at their highest in the Andean-Amazonian corridor, where the poverty level of informal rural households goes up to 68%, making their situation even worse due to the lack of rehab services and their isolation (Baker et al., 2020; Kay, 2018; Lindemann et al., 2025).

Informal settlements at urban peripheries, such as Mexico City, consist of disabled migrants coming from the countryside and needing help. In contrast, elderly rural informal workers are the most affected group (76% informality post-65), their condition being the blend of class poverty and racial exclusion from urban-centric policies. These divides serve as a political economy that allows disablement to subsidize cheap rural labor for export economies, thus continuing oppression (Duryea et al., 2019; OECD, 2025).

2.5 Structural Exclusion in Healthcare Systems

Structural exclusions in Latin America's healthcare, education, legal, and social systems, which define and limit people with disabilities based on race and class, even more so, are imposed on and thus burdensome to indigenous, Afro-descendant, and poor communities. These social systems are characterized by biomedical dominance, segregated schooling, uneven rights enforcement, and institutional neglect, which leads to the creation of obstacles that treat racialized bodies as pathological and, at the same time, prevent the emergence of decolonial alternatives. Nevertheless, grassroots resistance through mutual aid and pluriversal praxis offers many routes to disability justice, thereby challenging capitalist hierarchies.

Latin America's medical services are a perfect reflection of racialized capitalism as they focus on white man's medicine only, and at the same time, they create impossible barriers for the impoverished disabled people. Indigenous and Afro-descendants disabled people's needs are completely overlooked by public infrastructures that apply continuous underfunding and cultural erasure linked with class vulnerability (Garcia Mora et al., 2021; Rivas Velarde, 2022; Rodríguez Gatta et al., 2024; Rotarou & Sakellariou, 2017).

The biomedical model that is applied worldwide sees people with disabilities as sick people who need a cure through medical interventions. At the same time, indigenous worldviews are pushed back because they know the loss of abilities as something resulting from colonial oppression and environmental destruction. For instance, in Bolivia, the state medical clinics don't accept Aymara treatments and beliefs as scientific, and the Quechua disabled are forced to undergo treatments that are entirely different and neglect the spiritual aspect of health. This type of violence toward knowledge causes mental disabilities to worsen the suicide rates among indigenous people, being 2–3 times higher than the national rates in the midst of disrupted community healing networks. Afro-Honduran Garifuna people, who are also descendants of enslaved Africans, undergo a similar process of becoming invisible as the midwifery of their ancestors is replaced by hospital births, which cause more maternal ailments without any postpartum care (Lapierre, 2023; Reichenberger et al., 2024; Rivas Velarde, 2022; Rodríguez Gatta et al., 2024; Ullmann, 2016).

The access obstacles multiply this: disabled indigenous people in rural areas have to walk for days to clinics that are understaffed and do not have ramps, sign language, or Quechua interpreters, while Afro-Latinos in urban slums have to ration medicines that are beyond their informal incomes, which are 20–40% of the medicine prices. The affordability crisis is at its highest point in the privatized health care systems like Chile's, where social class divides give mestizo elites the privilege of accessing rehabilitation. At the same time, Mapuches suffer from untreated losses in their mobility as a result of logging injuries. The culturally unsafe care is reflected in the case of the Mayan communities in Guatemala, wherein the biomedical protocols ignore entirely the use of sweat lodge therapies leading to dropout rates of 50% and iatrogenic harms. The public health neglect during the COVID-19 pandemic exposed the racial fault lines—the Amazonian Yanomami were vaccinated weeks late, mercury poisoning from mining was not controlled, and this all contributed to the deterioration of the lives of people with disabilities by decades (Garcia Mora et al., 2021; Gatta et al., 2025; Reichenberger et al., 2024; Rodríguez Gatta et al., 2024; Rotarou & Sakellariou, 2017).

2.6 Educational Exclusion and Epistemic Injustice

Educational systems maintain these exclusions through narrative and linguistic erasure, thus stamping indigenous disabled pupils with the mark of epistemic injustice. Their knowledge is treated as inferior. The special education tracks racialize "deficits," pouring the racialized poor into the under-resourced silos that deny inclusive learning (Berlinski et al., 2021; Cantamutto & Costantino, 2023; Delprato, 2019; Lapierre, 2023).

Segregation continues despite the Salamanca Declaration promises, with 20–30% of disabled indigenous people being confined to special schools or totally excluded, just like the Quechua children in Peru's highlands who are diagnosed with autistic-like symptoms caused by cultural shyness. Racialized tracking in Brazil's favelas leads Afro-Brazilian disabled individuals to vocational dead-ends, while urban mestizos are given access to mainstream curricula. This sorting continues to cause disabled people to be illiterate, as the dropout rates of disabled indigenous students at the secondary level are as high as 60%. Language barriers are the leading cause of this illiteracy: Spanish-only assessments give a wrong diagnosis of the disabilities of 40 million indigenous speakers, cutting off the customization of support in the Mexican Nahuatl areas or the Colombian Wayuu territories. The rural-urban gap is another factor leading to this—informal kin carers in the Andes prioritize farm labor over schooling and silence literacy as a tool of epistemic power. Knowledge hierarchies silence the voices of disabled indigenous people by giving precedence to Western measurements over oral epistemologies. Mapuche stories of relational disability, where impairment is linked to the loss of territory, have no place in textbooks, thereby leaving students voiceless in policy discourses (Cantamutto & Costantino, 2023; Delprato, 2019; Duryea et al., 2019).

2.7 Legal Frameworks, Citizenship, and Unequal Protection

On-the-surface disability rights laws, though, progressive, offer unequal protection through patchy enforcement, criminalization, and racialized violence, which together deny citizenship to the most marginalized. CRPD ratification in Latin America and the Caribbean (LAC) leads to quotas and ramps that are not evenly realized, benefiting the urban formal sectors (Garcia Mora et al., 2021; Maciel et al., 2024; Rosado et al., 2025).

The implementation of disability laws varies across countries: Argentina's 26.378 law is of great help to residents of Buenos Aires but does nothing for the Guarani community in the province of Misiones; Ecuador's inclusion decree does not account for the isolation of people in the Amazon. Governments allocate only 0.5–1% of the budget to disability issues, suggesting that the indigenous clauses of ILO 169 are mere symbols amid the priority of extractive industries. Criminalization persecutes street-dwelling Afro-indigenous disabled individuals as vagrants, and those who are institutionalized are either put in asylums in Brazil or in psychiatric wards in Chile under the anti-vagrancy laws. Police violence during protests not only exacerbates the disability of the Mapuche community but is also protected by impunity, which is racialized and brutal. Access to justice is denied to the indigenous disabled population unless there are pro bono interpreters or adaptive courts; the rural Ixil in Guatemala rarely litigate their land-loss impairments, and Afro-Colombians are threatened by paramilitaries for making their claims (Duryea et al., 2019; Gatta et al., 2025; Lapierre, 2023; Rosado et al., 2025; UNICEF, 2015).

2.8 Resistance, Collective Agency, and Decolonial Futures

These practices challenge the biomedical and ableist states with pluriversal visions—oppression, grassroots movements create collective agency at disability-race-class intersections, and open the way to decolonial horizons through community care and solidarity economies. Confederations like Peru's CONADIS are positioned in the middle of the anti-mining front, where disabled indigenous people are at the forefront of the movement, blocking roads to reclaim their healing territories. Brazil's Unified Black Movement works with disability groups to create Afro-centric care centers that are a plus rather than a minus of institutionalization. Community-based care flourishes in Zapatista autonomous areas where Chiapas Maya share the costs of herbal clinics and peer rehab. They do this by going around the state that neglects them.

In Bolivia, solidarity economies created through cooperatives are engaging disabled Aymara people in the production of quinoa, which is integrated with a system of care that comes with the job. Decolonial practices envision disability in terms of Buen Vivir and follow indigenous cosmologies—Ecuador's Kichwa communities consider impairment a communal strength and demand government policies that reflect this through pluriversalism. Afro-Brazilian quilombos are extending mutual aid to disabled kin, thus demonstrating economies free of extraction. Such resistances are the start of a future with racial capitalism dismantled by disability justice, which would also ensure the amplification of the previously silenced voices in the harmony of territory-rooted worlds (Duryea et al., 2019; Gatta et al., 2025; Lapierre, 2023; Rivas Velarde, 2022; Rosado et al., 2025).

2.9 Conclusion

This chapter has argued that the issue of disability in Latin America should not be regarded as a marginal or secondary concern in intersectional analysis. However, it has to be acknowledged as a significant aspect of racially and class-based oppression that is very much rooted in colonial histories and current racialized capitalism. In all contexts such as extractive economies, informal labor markets, environmental racism, and structurally exclusionary institutions, disability is seen as both a result and a method of domination—created through unequal exposure to harm, denial of care, epistemic erasure, and unequal citizenship. When the chapter placed disability within the coloniality of power, knowledge, and being, an ableism phenomenon was shown to be operating alongside racism and class exploitation to build human hierarchies that made Indigenous, Afro-descendant, and poor bodies either disposable or invisible. Healthcare systems, educational institutions, and legal frameworks often reproduce these hierarchies by favoring Eurocentric, biomedical, and urban-centric norms while pushing community-based knowledges and practices to the periphery. These processes expose disability not as an individual flaw, but as a political and economic condition that is a result of historical dispossession and ongoing structural violence. Alongside this, the chapter has reaffirmed that oppressive situations are also sites of resistance. In Latin America, grassroots movements, solidarity economies, Indigenous cosmologies, and collective care practices are interrelated with the paradigms of reciprocity, relationality, and territoriality and, therefore, constitute pluralistic visions of disability, as they are not based on prevailing ableist and capitalist paradigms but instead offer new ones. These practices are envisioned as the prelude to decolonial futures, where disability justice will always be considered part of the struggle for land, dignity, epistemic recognition, and social transformation. The intersectional and decolonial frameworks that put disability at the center ultimately expand the scope of reimagining justice in Latin America, not only through the participation of disabled people in existing systems but also through the complete dismantling of the structures that give rise to inequalities.

References

Arbex, D. (2019). *Holocausto brasileiro*. Editora Intrinseca.

Artiga-Purcell, J. A., Chiasson-LeBel, T., Leiva, F., & Watanabe-Farro, A. (2023). Disaster extractivism: Latin America's extractive shock therapy in the age of COVID-19. *Latin American Perspectives, 50* (4), 172–192). https://doi.org/10.1177/0094582X231187886

Auz, J. (2024). The political ecology of climate remedies in Latin America and the Caribbean: Comparing compliance between national and inter-American litigation. *Journal of Human Rights Practice, 16*(1), 182–207. https://doi.org/10.1093/jhuman/huae007

Bachfischer, A., Barbosa, M. C., Rojas, A. A. R., Bechler, R., Schwienhorst-Stich, E. M., Kasang, C., et al. (2023). Implementing community based inclusive development for people with disability in Latin America: A mixed methods perspective on prioritized needs and lessons learned. *International Journal for Equity in Health, 22*(1), 147. https://doi.org/10.1186/s12939-023-01966-8

Baker, A., Berens, S., Feierherd, G., & González, I. M. (2020). Labor informality and its political consequences in Latin America. *Nashville: Latin American public opinion project.* Retrieved July 16, 2021, from https://doi.org/10.1017/lap.2022.4

Beard, S., Freeman, K., Velasco, M. L., Boyd, W., Chamberlain, T., Latoni, A., Lasko, D., Lunn, R. M., O'Fallon, L., Packenham, J., Smarr, M. M., Arnette, R., Cavalier-Keck, C., Keck, J., Muhammad, N., Wilson, O., Wilson, B., Wilson, A., & Dixon, D. (2024). Racism as a public health issue in environmental health disparities and environmental justice: Working toward solutions. *Environmental Health: A Global Access Science Source, 23*(1), 8. https://doi.org/10.1186/s12940-024-01052-8

Berlinski, S., Duryea, S., & Perez-Vincent, S. M. (2021). Prevalence and correlates of disability in Latin America and the Caribbean: Evidence from 8 national censuses. *PLoS One, 16*(10), e0258825. https://doi.org/10.1371/journal.pone.0258825

Cantamutto, F., & Costantino, A. (2023). Debt and the right to education in Latin America and the Caribbean. Feminism in public debt. A human right approach, 211–28. https://doi.org/10.56687/9781529237290-020

Choo, H. Y., & Ferree, M. M. (2010). Practicing intersectionality in sociological research: A critical analysis of inclusions, interactions, and institutions in the study of inequalities. *Sociological Theory, 28*(2), 129–149. https://doi.org/10.1111/j.1467-9558.2010.01370

Collins, P. H. (2000). *Black feminist thought: Knowledge, consciousness, and the politics of empowerment*. https://doi.org/10.4324/9780203900055

Collins, P. H., & Bilge, S. (2021). *Interseccionalidade*. Boitempo Editorial.

Curiel, O. (2020). *Construindo metodologias feministas a partir do feminismo decolonial. Pensamento feminista hoje: perspectivas decoloniais*. Bazar do Tempo.

Delprato, M. (2019). Parental education expectations and achievement for indigenous students in Latin America: Evidence from TERCE learning survey. *International Journal of Educational Development, 65*, 10–25. https://doi.org/10.1016/j.ijedudev.2018.12.004

Duryea, S., Salamanca, J. P. S., & Caicedo, M. P. (2019). *We the people: Inclusion of people with disabilities in Latin America and the Caribbean*. https://doi.org/10.18235/0002010

Féliz, M., & Melón, D. E. (2023). Beyond the green new deal? Dependency, racial capitalism and struggles for a radical ecological transition in Argentina and Latin America. *Geoforum, 145*, 103653. https://doi.org/10.1016/j.geoforum.2022.10.010

Fernández-Esquer, M. E., Aguerre, C. F., Ojeda, M., Brown, L. D., Atkinson, J. S., Rhoton, J. M., Da Silva, C. E., & Diamond, P. M. (2020). Documenting and understanding workplace injuries among Latino day laborers. *Journal of Health Care for the Poor and Underserved, 31*(2), 791–809. https://doi.org/10.1353/hpu.2020.0061

Ferrari, M. B. (2020). Feminismos descoloniales y discapacidad: hacia una conceptualización de la colonialidad de la capacidad. *Nómadas, 52*, 115–131. https://doi.org/10.30578/nomadas.n52a7

Frederick, A., & Shifrer, D. (2019). Race and disability: From analogy to intersectionality. *Sociology of Race and Ethnicity, 5*(2), 200–214. https://doi.org/10.1177/2332649218783480

Frederick, A. (2017). Risky mothers and the normalcy project: Women with disabilities negotiate scientific motherhood. *Gender & Society, 31*(1), 74–95. https://doi.org/10.1177/0891243216683914

Garcia Mora, M. E., Schwartz Orellana, S. D., & Freire, G. N. (2021). *Disability inclusion in Latin America and the Caribbean: A path to sustainable development.* https://hdl.handle.net/10986/36628

Gatta, D. R., Rotarou, E. S., Banks, L. M., & Kuper, H. (2025). Healthcare access among people with and without disabilities: A cross-sectional analysis of the National Socioeconomic Survey of Chile. *Public Health, 241*, 144–150. https://doi.org/10.1016/j.puhe.2025.02.010

Gerschick, T. J., & Stevens, J. D. (2016). Invisibility, visibility, vilification, and near silence: The framing of disability in the early years of the American sociological society. In *Sociology looking at disability: What did we know and when did we know it* (Vol. 9, pp. 1–27). Emerald Group Publishing Limited. https://doi.org/10.1108/S1479-354720160000009003

Gesser, M., Moraes, M. O., & Vale, G. M. D. S. M. D. (2024). Decolonizing ability, Latinizing feminist disability studies. *Revista Estudos Feministas, 32*, e101138. https://doi.org/10.1590/1806-9584-2024v32n3101138-en

Grosfoguel, R. (2016). A estrutura do conhecimento nas universidades ocidentalizadas: racismo/sexismo epistêmico e os quatro genocídios/epistemicídios do longo século XVI. *Sociedade e estado, 31*(1), 25–49. https://doi.org/10.1590/S0102-69922016000100003

Hammer, G. (2012). Blind women's appearance management: Negotiating normalcy between discipline and pleasure. *Gender & Society, 26*(3), 406–432. https://doi.org/10.1177/0891243212438263

Herrera, V. (2024). *Slow harms and citizen action: Environmental degradation and policy change in Latin American cities.* Oxford University Press. https://doi.org/10.1093/oso/9780197669020.001.0001

Iunes, R. F. (2002). *Occupational safety and health in Latin America and the Caribbean: Overview, issues and policy recommendations.* https://doi.org/10.18235/0008406

Kay, C. (2018). Rural Latin America: Exclusionary and uneven agricultural development. In *Capital, power, and inequality in Latin America* (pp. 21–52). Routledge. https://doi.org/10.4324/9780429501869-2

Lapierre, M. (2023). Disability and Latin American indigenous peoples. *Disability & Society, 38*(7), 1276–1280. https://doi.org/10.1080/09687599.2023.2192381

Lindemann, R., Yáñez, R., Cortínez, V., Carrasco, P., & Migueletto, C. (2025). *Latin American lessons on agroecology and territorial development to transition towards inclusive and climate-resilient food systems.* https://hdl.handle.net/10625/64538

Maciel, J. G., Del Valle, E., & Lutz, C. (2024). Health predictions in Latin America. *Journal of Insurance Medicine, 51*(1), 17–24. https://doi.org/10.17849/insm-51-1-17-24.1

Maroto, M., & Pettinicchio, D. (2015). Twenty-five years after the ADA: Situating disability in America's system of stratification. *Disability Studies Quarterly, 35*(3), 1–34. https://doi.org/10.18061/dsq.v35i3.4927

Mignolo, W. D. (2009). Epistemic disobedience, independent thought and decolonial freedom. *Theory, Culture & Society, 26*(7–8), 159–181. https://doi.org/10.1177/0263276409349275

Mignolo, W. D. (2017). Colonialidade: o lado mais escuro da modernidade. *Revista brasileira de ciências sociais, 32*, e329402. https://doi.org/10.17666/329402/2017

OECD. (2025). *Expanding social protection and addressing informality in Latin America.* OECD Publishing. https://doi.org/10.1787/86c1fd38-en

Phelan, J. C., Link, B. G., & Dovidio, J. F. (2008). Stigma and prejudice: One animal or two? *Social Science & Medicine, 67*(3), 358–367. https://doi.org/10.1016/j.socscimed.2008.03.022

Pucheta, M., & Kalil, R. (2025). Informal workers, vulnerability and human rights: An inter-American story. *Industrial Law Journal*, dwaf046. https://doi.org/10.1093/indlaw/dwaf046

Purfield, C. (2006). *Mind the gap-Is economic growth in India leaving some states behind?* https://doi.org/10.5089/9781451863635.001

Quijano, A. (2000). Colonialidad del poder y clasificación social. Festschrift for Immanuel Wallerstein. *Journal of World-Systems Research, VI*(2), 341–385. https://doi.org/10.5195/jwsr.2000.228

Quijano, A. (2005). *Colonialidade do poder, eurocentrismo e América Latina1. A Colonialidade do Saber: etnocentrismo e ciências sociais–Perspectivas Latinoamericanas* (pp. 107–126). Clacso. https://ria.ufrn.br/123456789/1661

Reed-Sandoval, A., & Sirvent, R. (2019). Disability and the decolonial turn: Perspectives from the Americas. *Disability and the Global South, 6*(1), 1553–1561.

Reichenberger, V., Corona, A. P., Ramos, V. D., Shakespeare, T., Hameed, S., Penn-Kekana, L., & Kuper, H. (2024). Access to primary healthcare services for adults with disabilities in Latin America and the Caribbean: A review and meta-synthesis of qualitative studies. *Disability and Rehabilitation, 46*(25), 6011–6020. https://doi.org/10.1080/09638288.2024.2320268

Rivas Velarde, M. (2022). 566 indigenous perspectives on disability. In *The Oxford handbook of the sociology of disability* (pp. 566–582). Oxford University Press. https://doi.org/10.1093/oxfordhb/9780190093167.013.33

Robeyns, I. (2025). *Pluralizing political philosophy: Economic and ecological inequalities in global perspective* (p. 352). Oxford University Press. https://doi.org/10.1093/9780191994784.003.0011

Rodríguez Aguilera, M. Y. (2021). Everyday resistances to environmental racism, mestizo geographies, and toxicity in Oaxaca. *The Funambulist Magazine.*

Rodríguez Gatta, D., Rotenberg, S., Allel, K., Reichenberger, V., Banks, L. M., & Kuper, H. (2024). Access to general health care among people with disabilities in Latin America and the Caribbean: A systematic review of quantitative research. *Lancet Regional Health. Americas, 32*, 100701. https://doi.org/10.1016/j.lana.2024.100701

Rosado, C. B. F., Chura-Quispe, G., Herrera-Pérez, E. I., Vargas-Murillo, A. R., Collazos-Alarcón, M. A., & Alatrista-Vargas, E. A. (2025). Violence against persons with disabilities in Latin America: A systematic review. *Multidisciplinary Reviews, 9*(6), 2026257. https://doi.org/10.31893/multirev.2026257

Rotarou, E. S., & Sakellariou, D. (2017). Inequalities in access to health care for people with disabilities in Chile: The limits of universal health coverage. *Critical Public Health, 27*(5), 604–616. https://doi.org/10.1080/09581596.2016.1275524

Ruiz-Negrón, B., Lemus, A., Echeverri Herrera, S., Tovar, A., Arreola, A., Hess, J. M., & Goodkind, J. R. (2026). The work-wellbeing paradox: Exploring the emotional and bodily dimensions of intersectional capitalism among Latinx immigrants in the U.S. *Social Science & Medicine, 388*, 118747. https://doi.org/10.1016/j.socscimed.2025.118747

Silva, R. P. D. (2011). *Uma genealogia de infames.* https://doi.org/10.1590/S1415-47142011000100014

Stlouka, L., SNELL, C. J., & Koob, A. (2024). *Disability and development report 2024: Accelerating the realization of the sustainable development goals by, for and with persons with disabilities.* https://social.desa.un.org/sites/default/files/inline-files/Goal8.pdf

Telles, E. E., Bailey, S. R., Davoudpour, S., & Freeman, N. C. (2025). Racial inequality in Latin America. *Oxford Open Economics, 4*(Supplement_1), i200–i218. doi:https://doi.org/10.1093/ooec/odae022.

Ullmann, H. (2016). Health and young people in Latin America and the Caribbean. *Youth: Realities and Challenges for Achieving Development with Equality, 63.*

UNICEF, (2015). *Advancement of the UN CRPD through the 2030 agenda towards implementation in Latin America.* https://www.internationaldisabilityalliance.org/sites/default/files/documents/final_lac_report.pdf

Utzet, M., Botías, F., Silva-Peñaherrera, M., Tobías, A., & Benavides, F. G. (2021). Informal employment and poor self-perceived health in Latin America and the Caribbean: A gender-based comparison between countries and welfare states in a pooled analysis of 176,786 workers. *Globalization and Health, 17*(1), 140. https://doi.org/10.1186/s12992-021-00792-3

Chapter 3
Embodiment, Relationality, and Difference in Indigenous Worldviews

Abstract Disability is one of the issues addressed in this chapter through the lenses of Indigenous worldviews in Latin America. These civilizations embody, relate, and differ through the nature of their culture and history. For instance, in the West, the concept of disability has been associated with the biomedical and neoliberal models that view it as a matter of personal problem, thus limiting the discourse to the individual's deficit, autonomy, and productivity. The chapter, however, places disability within collective world's perspectives where kin, land, faith, and reciprocity define the existence. Based on decoloniality theory, Southern ways of knowing and Indigenous concepts, it shows that colonization, exploitation, political repression, and forced assimilation have not only marginalized Indigenous peoples but have also rendered them epistemically disabled. In this way, the chapter through the application of concepts such as diálogo de saberes, Buen Vivir, and relational ontologies portrays disability as a natural and a shared social responsibility rather than a deviation from the normative function. The Indigenous ways of caring, working, and being involved focus more on interdependence and moral obligation than on the market's productivity, thus providing different avenues for inclusion and resistance. In recognition of the importance of Indigenous-led research practices and activism, the chapter proposes a re-examination of the field of disability studies that will be multi-national, cross-cultural, and diverse in terms of knowledge, and thus, able to tackle the persistent colonial conditions affecting disability in the Global South.

Keywords Indigenous disability · Coloniality · Rationality · Decolonization and Latin America

3.1 Introduction

Disability is a common occurrence among the indigenous peoples of Latin America and has some specific features attached to it. On one hand, the people involved have their own particular understanding and feelings about disabilities, which are influenced by their worldviews and cultural practices; on the other hand, these cultural

S. M. Thomas and R. Veerabathiran, *Disability and Decolonial Thought in Latin America*, SpringerBriefs in Modern Perspectives on Disability Research,
https://doi.org/10.1007/978-981-95-8950-0_3

characteristics are partly the result of a disability that has been inflicted by colonialism, colonization, and forced assimilation to the states. Moreover, the living conditions of the indigenous peoples which are economically poor, together with the political violence against them, make the situation so complex that it becomes a challenge for disability studies to collaborate with other philosophical disciplines. Decoloniality, interculturality, epistemologies of the South, and indigenous thought can be seen as avenues through which the study of disability in indigenous cultures can be more fairly and contextually viewed and also one that would cause rather than avoid relevant issues (Lapierre, 2023).

Certain research has verified that the disabled population among the indigenous is greater than that among the non-indigenous. The United Nations (2013) duly noted that this is the case in the countries of Australia, New Zealand, Canada, Costa Rica, Ecuador, Mexico, Panama, and Uruguay. In Chile, the same scenario has been established for the case of children and young people (National Disability Service, 2016). In indigenous communities, disability is not only theologically, but also philosophically and sociologically determined, through the cultural lens, including the history of their ancestors (Meekosha, 2011). Many don't even have a term in their mother language to signify disability, whereas some have even traced it back to the very beginnings of their myths (Yarza de los Ríos & Romualdo Pérez, 2021). These odd cultural traits are still part of the whole picture of a disability caused by the process of colonization and conquest (Grech & Soldatic, 2015). But they also are the very circumstances like extreme poverty, intra-regional migration, globalization, the economic power of North countries, the consequences of recent military dictatorships, the impact of the Spanish conquest on the native indigenous peoples of today's Latin America, internal colonialism, and the political violence of states against these peoples. In the last decades, however, the growing neoliberalism led to the states' implementation of intercultural health programs that were more of a moneymaking venture for the states than a genuine interculturality that was really, as Boccara (2012) and Vicente Marín & Gil García, 2017 said, a battlefield.

Furthermore, it can be pointed out that some Latin American countries have adopted the social model of disability but in a manner that has resulted in weak, confused, and accommodated applications of the model, which may be far from the strong social, critical, and political principles that are the basis of the model. Besides this, native people have their own knowledge systems that not only give them insights about their being and living but also include their understanding of disability. This situation prompts the disability studies to work in deeper dialogues with other philosophies that native people consider more just for them. These theoretical encounters will lead to the creation of reciprocal intercultural knowledge and practices showing that disability is a heterogeneous, plurinational, and epistemically diverse territory (Lapierre, 2023).

In this context, disability is perceived as an Indigenous worldviews' stigmas that highlight the discourse of collective existence by affirming the bodies' and their relationships' differences instead of focusing on the individual impairments. Pre-Columbian peoples of the Americas showed that the idea of disability depended on a web of connections among bodies, communities, land, ancestors, and gods, thus providing views that contest the prevailing medical and state-centered models. The application of decolonial thinking, Southern epistemologies, and indigenous philosophies leads to an incisive questioning of how much colonial brutality, neoliberal governance, and only skin-deep intercultural policy have affected the modern-day disability conditions, usually at the cost of the marginalization of the native knowledge systems. In contrast, an indigenous viewpoint might define disability as a multitude of plurals and ethnicities that are united through care, moral duty and are in close contact with the ancestral wisdom. The chapter thereby significantly enriches the disability field by unveiling these diverse perspectives and through the promotion of an intercultural and relational viewpoint that regards pagan ways of knowing as the most meaningful sources of theory, practice, and resistance.

3.2 Decolonizing Disability with Indigenous Peoples Research in Latin America

The identification of indigenous peoples as socio-economically disadvantaged has been one of the main paths through which the Latin American states have interacted with the disability issue among the indigenous peoples. This has led to the recognition of these populations as doubly vulnerable, and a series of state actions have emerged that are based on this perspective of difference and, thus, the ongoing debates regarding the social disadvantages. Some of these actions are disability pensions, training for informal caregivers, economic benefits, support for entrepreneurship, etc. However, the disadvantage of being socially excluded is a reality, and many of these actions are indeed necessary and demanded by the people themselves, still state subsidiarity fails to question the causes of this disadvantage and also does not problematize the historical role of the state in this causality. In this regard, states prefer to turn a blind eye to the structures that characterize modern colonialism and to the relations of dominance, hierarchy, and hegemony among the ethnic groups. They also create a condition of economic dependence with the indigenous peoples, thereby controlling and dominating the conflicts with the natives that the modern nation-states have in their territories. The recent consultation with the Mapuche people in Chile conducted by the Constitutional Convention highlights this issue. The Mapuche people thought it was necessary for the interdiction of disabled persons to continue to be legalized in order for the family to receive the economic benefits, while at the same time supporting the autonomy of disabled indigenous persons (Castillo Valdivia & Tapia Cuevas, 2025; Lapierre, 2023). Such a paradox is not strange as it is also the case that in subsidiary economies, it is seen as a consequence of the historical marginalization of the peoples and their economic dependence on the state.

Disability, as a social phenomenon, should be placed with a corresponding cultural establishment of its particularities. This opens a way to dialogue among various schools of thought, which is called diálogo desaberes (this is dialogue between different systems of beliefs and knowledge, rationalities, and traditions) (Leff, 2013).

Intercultural health and social bearing the use of different equally ranked belief systems through the dialogue can relate aspects of the worldview. It may also initiate and promote research projects on disability and aboriginal that are based on each nation's own methodology—that is, not as essentialist but as situated and thus understanding them. Since the diálogo de saberes is conducted under ethical, fair, and equitable conditions, it can be expected that the knowledge and practices of indigenous people within the field of disability will be able to cross the boundaries of non-indigenous society and not just the other way around. Hence, disability studies or crip theory may be "shaken" by the philosophies and methodologies of the native peoples of Abya Yala (this is the name that indigenous peoples prefer for the American continent, since it recovers a traditional way of naming it, used by the Kuna people before the arrival of Columbus. It is translated as "land in vital blood") (Del Popolo, 2017). This signifies that, for instance, indigenous ontologies and epistemologies, along with their life practices, could be both a theoretical and practical point of reference tore fresh and rethink the significance of and impact that disability studies have in Latin America and other areas of the Global South. Hence, indigenous struggles, social demands, and worldviews ought to be part and parcel of disability studies rather than simply a challenge or complementary.

Moreover, the disability professionals dealing with indigenous peoples should be in the frontline of the indigenous activism, as their contribution will be toward the practices of resistance that the peoples and the collectives undertake. This means that both the health professionals and the scholars become activists and support the indigenous resistance. The struggles that are faced are not only in the domain of health, disability, or inclusion, since the indigenous worldviews are grounded on the complex concept of Buen Vivir (concept proposed by Latin American indigenous peoples as an alternative to the concept of development, based on principles of reciprocity, community, and harmony with nature) (Del Popolo, 2017). Thus, disability activism can easily be transferred to other domains like land recovery, protection of sacred territories for ancestral medicine, environmental care, language revitalization, etc., since these issues are all interrelated and bear great significance for the well living models that characterize the peoples of Abya Yala.

The growing number of indigenous movements in Latin America has made it evident that the common struggle mainly consists in acknowledgment as peoples that existed before, that are still alive and that have legitimate demands; and with this, the right to live as a nation, to keep the language, to get back their usurped lands, to have self-determination and autonomy. Besides these, there are other more specific demands concerning health, education, or the environment, which are the basis of the main movement. In Latin America, though they are few in number, there are some leaders or groups of indigenous people with disabilities who have built up an interesting discourse, experience, and history on disability that goes against the prevailing models of approach. The discourse on disability can be found also in the demands related to the protection of sacred territories for the practice of ancestral medicine or to the issue of environmental pollution. These struggles are at once ecological, cultural, medicinal, spiritual, and ethical (Lapierre, 2023).

There exist pioneering research practices in Latin America that can be seen as a part of a critical interculturality (Walsh, 2010) and that are framed within an accumulation of the decolonial, feminist and intercultural perspectives that manage to combine socio-historical and contemporary critical ethnographic studies of disability (Lapierre, 2022; Moctezuma Balderas, 2020; Yarza de los Ríos & Romualdo Pérez, 2021). These research problems might be tackled only through a process of decolonization of the researchers and practitioners who would come to interpret disability in indigenous peoples from such a perspective that is at the frontiers and would be accompanied by the common struggles of the peoples, modernly-colonially impacted by the world system, and thus sharing the same struggles with the frontiers. The very first and probably the toughest challenge is to push for studies that portray and present the non-western world through their spirituality, culture and diversity of the indigenous world in terms of disability in parallel to an impact and a research that can appropriately complicate the phenomenon of disability at a historical juncture where indigenous peoples are under threat and disability is also caused by such harshness as colonialism, environmental extractivism, and systematic violence. Forging political and militant research that empowers the indigenous people and equips them with the tools for their struggles is of utmost importance today. Ultimately, even if some indigenous languages will be lost due to racism and forced assimilation, the cultural experience of disability will never be accessible even if the entire Spanish language is there to communicate. Language holds the knowledge and it flows to the next generation through it. Hence, linguistic loss means knowledge loss.

3.3 Disability: Variation, Reciprocity, and Interdependence

Through relational ontologies that refuse Western deficit models, Indigenous thought in Latin America reconsider's ability, difference, and disability. As a result, disability is seen as a natural variation among the community, not a tragic impairment, which is, however, supported by reciprocity and oral narratives that give meaning to embodied difference. These worldviews oppose the colonial individualism and place care as a collective responsibility that is linked to both territory and ancestors.

Esoteric thoughts of Native peoples throughout the Latin American continent view human potential as something that flows and varies with the circumstances, and comes from dealings instead of being a trait of the individual. The concept of difference, regardless if it is physical, cognitive, or sensory, is considered a source of life diversity among the community and not a reason for classification or shortage. This connection-based outlook, which can be seen in Andean ayllu and Amazonian shamanism, treats human differences as similes of ecological variety where every being plays a role in the flourishing of the whole (Lapierre, 2023; Rivas Velarde, 2022).

In Quechua culture, disability terms such as "llaki" (sorrowful imbalance) signify a temporary state of disbalance which can be restored through ritual reciprocity, not a permanent loss. The same way Mayan ontologies picture impairments as "k'ax k'ay" (twisted sight), a change in perception which shows previously obscured worlds, and not blindness as a loss of vision. The Mapuche have the word "weyla" which covers bodily differences as the marks of the spirit giving the person resilience and thus opposing the biomedical tragedy narratives. These cultural frames place variance as a source of life; the deaf elders in Guarani communities, for instance, act as intuitive mediators with the non-human realms because their sensory profiles add to the group wisdom rather than being a burden (Gurung, 2022; Lapierre, 2023).

This is in sharp contrast to the models of settlers: colonial missions regarded the indigenous body's manifestations as diseases, declining shamanic trance, and labeling it as madness or considering albinism among Taino people as demonic. The present-day violence of extraction is creating "new" disabilities, such as mercury-induced trembling of the Yanomami—but still, the indigenous people respond by reintegrating them as the territorial wounds that are demanding communal repair, not individual curing (Velarde, 2018).

Reciprocity perceives care as a two-way street system, where the disabled family members get the assistance, they need and at the same time are contributing through prophecy, memory-keeping, or craft. In Aymara communities in Bolivia, disabled weavers teach the little ones how to read patterns and their slow-moving hands are imparting the patience that is considered the very knowledge. This action eliminates the division between caregiver and care-receiver and integrates care within the daily gatherings where absence (e.g., migration for wage labor) is more disruptive to harmony than bodily difference (Gurung, 2022; Lapierre, 2023).

The whole community has a responsibility not only in the care but also in the prevention: Tzotzil rituals strengthen and protect the pregnant women from the imbalance, and at the same time, the society views the disability precursors as communal alerts to social discord. In the times of crisis like droughts, the disabled elders are the ones deciding where the resources are going, and their immobility symbolizes being rooted in the center of the change (Velarde, 2018).

Interdependence is a multiverse concept that explains the link of human disabilities to past due taxes, future crops, and the cycle of time and space. In the Shuar tribe in Ecuador, difficulties in moving indicate the calling of the forest for the return of the tree; thus, human bodies are tied to the spirits of the jaguar and the flow of the river. The land is even related to people: in Nahua stories, paralyzed bodies "hold the milpa," thus stabilizing the soil through their immobility while mobile relatives are wearing out the soil, thereby overturning ableist notions of productivity (Duryea et al., 2019; Lapierre, 2023).

Even more, non-human relations add to this—deaf Wayuu herdsmen are remarkably perceptive of camelid vibrations, they are the ones who feed the herd better than the hearing people, as their world of senses is the best support for the flock. The webs of generations twist and turn but guarantee the supply: grand-parents suffering from dementia are able to recall the songs of their people, their slow and unclear speaking is the hint for the young to embody them through movement (Gurung, 2022).

3.4 Contrasts with Western Norms of Autonomy and Productivity

The Western understanding of disability and the body is very much influenced by the philosophical roots that consider individualism, freedom, and productivity as the main criteria of one's value. It is the liberal and neoliberal societies that create the image of an ideal person who is self-controlled, economically productive, and physically and mentally efficient. Bodies that do not conform to these norms are most often perceived as deficient or dependent and thus the prevalence of ableism that places non-normative bodies at the margins is reinforced (Davis, 1997, 2016; Lovern & Locust, 2013). The Indigenous peoples' view of the world, on the other hand, greatly differs from this by promoting the notion of relationships and community duties and thus indirectly disputing the generalization of Western autonomy-based models. Table 3.1 depicts the Western Autonomy–Productivity Norms versus Indigenous Relational Models in Disability.

Individualism in the West draws its historical background from the Enlightenment that emphasized the character of a person based on rational independence and self-sufficiency. While people who are dependent on others are often seen as morally lacking or simply taking a temporary break from being adults, such a mindset spreads over the legal, medical, and social welfare systems where the idea of independence is viewed as being dignified and of social value (Davis, 1997; Markus & Kitayama, 1998). Lovern (2017) mentions these constructions as being culturally specific and not universal. He also points out that they can be very disruptive when they are applied to Indigenous people's ways of life since they have been acknowledging interdependence as a basic human condition for a long time through their relational systems.

The capitalist economies of the world make the situation more complicated by attaching the value of a person's body to his or her labor effectiveness and output. The body is trained and optimized like a machine and judged by its ability to perform up to the standards of the different types of work: industrial and post-industrial. People whose bodies or minds do not meet the set standards for being productive are pushed to the edges of the economy and the society where they are not even noticed (Bell, 2010; Davis, 2016). Lovern (2017) believes that this reasoning is the root of contemporary disability discrimination, which makes the difference seem like a deficiency instead of being a legitimate form of human diversity.

Indigenous ways of knowing basically turn the idea of self-sufficiency upside down by putting interdependence and relational identity at the forefront. The individual is viewed not as independent but rather as being made up of the relationships with his/her/their family, community, land, ancestors, and even non-human beings. Dependence is not seen as something bad but rather as a fact admitting to life's inevitable and cyclical nature which different people go through at different times (Cajete, 2000; Lovern, 2017; Manuka, 2001). When viewed from this angle, Western autonomy is recognized as a limited cultural notion that hides the relations which are the most basic foundations of human existence.

Table 3.1 Western autonomy–productivity norms versus indigenous relational models in disability

Core theme	Western autonomy & productivity framework	Indigenous relational framework	Specific consequences for disabled persons	Policy implications	Key references
Basis of human value	Human worth tied to independence and economic output	Human worth grounded in relational belonging	Disabled persons devalued under productivity norms	Policies must decouple human value from economic productivity	Davis (1997); Lovern (2017)
Meaning of autonomy	Autonomy defined as self-sufficiency	Autonomy embedded in interdependence	Dependency stigmatized vs normalized	Inclusion policies should recognize interdependence as legitimate autonomy	Lovern (2017); Markus and Kitayama (1998)
View of dependency	Dependency viewed as moral or social deficit	Dependency accepted as cyclical and shared	Welfare surveillance and stigma	Social protection systems should move away from deficit-based eligibility criteria	Cajete (2000); Davis (1997)
Productivity standard	Standardized labor output defines social contribution	Contribution defined through relational roles	Exclusion from labor-based inclusion schemes	Disability policies must broaden definitions of productivity	Davis (2016); Bell (2010)
Definition of work	Paid employment prioritized	Care, ritual, healing, and cultural labor recognized	Unpaid contributions rendered invisible	Policies should formally recognize and support non-market labor	Cajete (2000); Lovern (2017)
Treatment of non-conforming bodies	Bodies failing efficiency norms labeled deficient	Bodily difference accepted as diversity	Increased medicalization and stigma	Health and education policies should adopt strengths-based approaches	Lovern (2017); Wendell (1989)
Normal / abnormal distinction	Central organizing binary	Largely absent	Reinforcement of ableist classifications	Disability assessment systems should avoid rigid functional hierarchies	Waters (2008)

(continued)

Table 3.1 (continued)

Core theme	Western autonomy & productivity framework	Indigenous relational framework	Specific consequences for disabled persons	Policy implications	Key references
Medicalization of disability	Disability framed as individual pathology	Disability understood as relational condition	Focus on cure rather than participation	Shift policy focus from cure-oriented to participation-oriented models	Davis (2016); Lovern (2017)
Citizenship criteria	Citizenship linked to labor participation	Citizenship linked to belonging and reciprocity	Exclusion from civic legitimacy	Redefine citizenship rights beyond employment status	Davis (1997); Morgensen (2011)
Assessment and surveillance	Proof of incapacity required for support	Community recognition of needs	Deficit-based identities reinforced	Reform welfare assessments to reduce surveillance and stigma	Davis (2016); Lovern (2017)
Flexibility of social roles	Rigid role expectations	Roles adapted to capacities	Loss of participation opportunities	Policies should allow flexible participation pathways	Manuka (2001); Montejo (2001)
Concept of inclusion	Inclusion equated with labor-market integration	Inclusion defined as relational participation	Narrow inclusion outcomes	Inclusion policies must move beyond employment-only metrics	Gilley (2011); Lovern (2017)
Global Disability & Development Agendas	Export Western productivity norms	Indigenous relational values marginalized	Reproduction of colonial ableism	International frameworks must be culturally adaptable	Lovern (2017); UN (2007)
Source of disability marginalization	Individual incapacity emphasized	Colonial disruption of relational systems highlighted	Structural causes obscured	Policies must address historical and structural determinants	Deloria (2006); Echo-Hawk (2016)

(continued)

Table 3.1 (continued)

Core theme	Western autonomy & productivity framework	Indigenous relational framework	Specific consequences for disabled persons	Policy implications	Key references
Response to disability exclusion	Individual rehabilitation and self-management	Collective and community-based care	Isolation vs collective support	Support community-led and indigenous-driven disability initiatives	Lovern (2017)
Overall effect on disabled lives	Marginalization, monitoring, exclusion	Recognition, participation, dignity	Disability seen as deficit vs diversity	Policy paradigms must align with decolonial disability justice	Davis (2016); Lovern (2017)

Many Indigenous peoples' cultures do not use functional norms to rank bodies. They are not medicalized or moralized but accepted as a natural aspect of diversity. The "normal/abnormal" dichotomy is absent in the case of Indigenous peoples and illustrates their non-dualistic epistemologies which oppose the ranking of people on the basis of perfection or efficiency ideals (Lovern, 2017; Waters, 2008; Wendell, 1989). These frameworks have made it possible for people with different kinds of bodies or minds to continue participating fully in social and cultural life.

In Western contexts, productivity is not simply a matter of economic necessity; it is also a moral duty that is closely linked with the concepts of citizenship and social legitimacy. Those who are not able to dedicate themselves to full-time or standardized work are usually put under scrutiny by means of medical and welfare systems that require constant proof of incapacity, which in turn, gives rise to and strengthens deficit-based identities (Davis, 1997; Davis, 2016). Lovern (2017) offers an example of how these mechanisms subject Indigenous people with disabilities to the imposition of standards of labor value that are externally defined and which contradict with Indigenous peoples' ways of contributing.

In Indigenous societies, contribution is seen in the context of relationships and not of economic transactions. Caregiving, storytelling, ritual participation, healing practices, and cultural transmission are some examples of activities that are none the less considered essential forms of labor even when they do not bring in any money. The measure of a person's contribution is done according to his/her abilities and talents and not through the application of abstract productivity norms (Cajete, 2000; Lovern, 2017). This strengths-based approach does not allow for the exclusion of non-normative bodies and it also acknowledges the social value of all community members.

Flexibility in roles is another aspect that makes Indigenous practices of embodiment and labor different from others. People with physical or mental differences are not only allowed to participate but are also to do so in a manner that corresponds to their capabilities. These customs reveal a community spirit where the burden of responsibility is not uniformly imposed but rather shared and adjusted (Lovern, 2017; Manuka, 2001; Montejo, 2001). This stands in stark contrast to the Western systems which more or less require the conformity of the body to the norms of the society as a condition for being accepted.

At the same time, globalization of exclusion on the ground of disabilities in development is one of the main issues in international disability and development frameworks. Such agendas often repeat the Western productivity norms by placing the emphasis on employment, independence, self-management, and so on, making them the ultimate road to empowerment. As progressive these models are proclaimed to be, they run the risk of extending coloniality to Indigenous peoples due to their prioritization of the market over relations (Lovern, 2017; UN, 2007).

The idea of Indigenous relationality reveals the presence of the neoliberal inclusion's limitations and, consequently, it redefines participation as a relational engagement instead of an economic assimilation. To an Indigenous person, Inclusion means the existence of relationships that not only keep the group but also maintain its balance and well-being. When the policies for inclusion turn their back on this relational base, they not only risk undermining the Indigenous knowledge systems, but also sealing the fate of the existing societal divisions (Gilley, 2011; Lovern, 2017; Morgensen, 2011).

Indigenous scholars, in particular, point out that the marginalization of the disabled is grounded in the wider context of colonization, displacement, and processes of poverty that have been institutionalized. They equate the disabled with the unfit in society and, hence, push them to the periphery of social circles. As a result, the collective nature and decolonization processes rather than the individualized, productivity or self-sufficiency-based solutions are what the deaf need (Deloria, 2006; Echo-Hawk, 2016; Lovern, 2017).

Thus, the discrepancy between Indigenous relational epistemologies and the Western norms of autonomy and productivity discloses disability as a category produced by culture rather than a universal state. The Indigenous worldviews bring to light the prevailing notions concerning the concepts of labor, independence, and human value; at the same time, they provide alternative embodiments of inclusion rooted in reciprocity, interdependence, and respect for embodied differences.

3.5 Conclusion

The chapter has presented an argument that disability within the Indigenous peoples of Latin America cannot be comprehended properly if one uses the universal Western models based on autonomy, independence, and productivity. On the contrary, the Indigenous perspectives define disability as a type of relational difference that is incarnate in the networks of community, land, ancestry, and spirituality. These perspectives not only challenge but also redefine the existing narratives of disability that are based on the view of the disabled as less fortunate, by representing the disabled persons as being in difficult but healthy and equal relations with others. They do this through claiming that the disabled are not the only ones who give, but also through the operation of moral and social responsibilities, and then sharing the collective care where interdependence is not a limiting factor but rather the most basic life condition. The chapter situates disability in the context of colonization, forced assimilation, environmental abuse, and neoliberal governance, thus showing that many present-day disabilities are more a consequence of social systems than of individual cases. Inclusion policies by states and social models of disability when alienated from Indigenous knowledge systems, could very well be the ones driving the same old colonial hierarchies and economic dependencies. The chapter advocates that disability studies should not only be about those who are disabled but rather be a militant, anti-colonial, and Indigenous-led research, and practice. Seeing disability as a diverse, multi-national, and epistemically rich domain opens up the possibility for fairer and more context-sensitive perceiving of body and difference. This manner of dealing with the subject not only strengthens disability theory but also brings scholarship into the fold of Indigenous struggles for self-determination, land, cultural survival, and collective well-being in Latin America and the Global South.

References

Bell, C. (2010). Is disability studies actually white disability studies. *The disability studies reader, 5*, 402–410. https://doi.org/10.4324/9781315680668-38

Boccara, G. (2012). La interculturalidad como campo social. *Cuadernos interculturales, 10*(18), 11–30. http://www.redalyc.org/articulo.oa?id=55223841002

Cajete, G. (2000). Little Bear, L. Native science: Natural laws of interdependence.

Castillo Valdivia, N. G., & Tapia Cuevas, L. A. M. (2025). *El proceso de consulta indígena en la estrategia nacional del litio en Chile.* https://doi.org/10.58011/pgzp-t697.

Davis, L. J. (1997). Constructing normalcy. *The Disability Studies Reader, 3*, 3–19.

Davis, L. J. (2016). *The disability studies reader.* Routledge. https://doi.org/10.4324/9781315680668

Del Popolo, F. (2017). *Los pueblos indígenas en América (Abya Yala).* CLACSO.

Deloria, V. (2006). *The world we used to live in: Remembering the powers of the medicine men.* Fulcrum Publishing.

Duryea, S., Salamanca, J. P. S., & Caicedo, M. P. (2019).*We the people: Inclusion of people with disabilities in Latin America and the Caribbean.* https://doi.org/10.18235/0002010

Echo-Hawk, W. R. (2016). *In the light of justice: The rise of human rights in native America and the UN declaration on the rights of indigenous peoples.* Fulcrum Publishing. https://doi.org/10.5860/choice.51-2930

Gilley, B. J. (2011). Two-Spirit men's sexual survivance against the inequality of desire. *Queer indigenous studies: Critical interventions in theory, politics, and literature*, 123–31.

Grech, S., & Soldatic, K. (2015). Disability and colonialism:(dis) encounters and anxious intersectionalities. *Social Identities, 21*(1), 1–5. https://doi.org/10.1080/13504630.2014.995394

Gurung, P. (2022). *Indigenous persons with disabilities global network (IPWDGN).* Indigenous World.

Lapierre, M. (2022). Caracterización sociodemográfica de la prevalencia de discapacidad en la población indígena de Chile. *Revista Chilena de Salud Pública, 26*(2), 203–213. https://doi.org/10.5354/0719-5281.2022.71206

Lapierre, M. (2023). Disability and Latin American indigenous peoples. *Disability & society, 38*(7), 1276–1280. https://doi.org/10.1080/09687599.2023.2192381

Leff, E. (2013). *Aventuras de la Epistemología Ambiental: De la articulación de Ciencias al Diálogo de Saberes.* Siglo XXI Editores México.

Lovern, L., & Locust, C. (2013). *Native American communities on health and disability: A borderland dialogues.* Spring. https://doi.org/10.1057/9781137312020

Lovern, L. L. (2017). Indigenous perspectives on difference: A case for inclusion. *Journal of Literary & Cultural Disability Studies, 11*(3), 303–320. https://doi.org/10.3828/jlcds.2017.24

Manuka, H. (2001). Tapu, Mana, Mauri, Hau, Wairua: A Maori philosophy of vitalism and cosmos. *Indigenous Traditions and Ecology*, 197–221. https://doi.org/10.1108/978-1-68123-157-020251009

Markus, H. R., & Kitayama, S. (1998). The cultural psychology of personality. *Journal of Cross-Cultural Psychology, 29*(1), 63–87. https://doi.org/10.1177/0022022198291004

Meekosha, H. (2011). Decolonising disability: Thinking and acting globally. *Disability & Society, 26*(6), 667–682. https://doi.org/10.1080/09687599.2011.602860

Moctezuma Balderas, A. C. (2020). El trabajo de cuidados de la infancia nahua con discapacidad. El caso de las madres de la Huasteca potosina, México. *Revista de El Colegio de San Luis, 10*(21) https://doi.org/10.21696/rcs1102120201246

Montejo, V. D. (2001). The road to heaven: Jakaltek Maya beliefs, religion, and the ecology. *Indigenous traditions and ecology: The interbeing of cosmology and community*, (pp. 175–95). https://doi.org/10.5860/choice.39-3466

Morgensen, S. L. (2011). Unsettling queer politics. *Queer indigenous studies: Critical interventions in theory, politics, and literature*, (pp. 132–152).

Rivas Velarde, M. (2022). 566 indigenous perspectives on disability. In *The Oxford handbook of the sociology of disability* (pp. 566–582). Oxford University Press. https://doi.org/10.1093/oxfordhb/9780190093167.013.33

United Nations. General Assembly. (2007). Convention on the rights of persons with disabilities and optional protocol. *UN*.

Velarde, M. R. (2018). Indigenous perspectives of disability. *Disability Studies Quarterly, 38*(4). https://doi.org/10.1093/oxfordhb/9780190093167.013.33

Vicente Marín, P., & Gil García, F. (2017). Interculturalidad en salud. Dudas, limitaciones y repliegues. In *Medicinas y cuerpos en América Latina: debates antropológicos desde la salud y la interculturalidad* (pp. 53–98). Editorial Universitaria Abya Yala.

Walsh, C. (2010). Interculturalidad crítica y educación intercultural. *Construyendo interculturalidad crítica, 75*(96), 167–181.

Waters, A. (2008). *American Indian thought: Philosophical essays*. https://doi.org/10.2979/TRANCHARPEIRSOC.54.2.09

Wendell, S. (1989). Toward a feminist theory of disability. *Hypatia, 4*(2), 104–124. https://doi.org/10.1111/j.1527-2001.1989.tb00576.x

Yarza de los Ríos, A., & Romualdo Pérez, Z. (2021). Discapacidad desde y en los pueblos indígenas en Abya Yala/Afro/Latino/América: Aproximaciones desde Colombia (mundo Êbêra Eyábida) y México (mundo Ayüük Jääy). *P. Danel; B. Pérez Ramírez; y A. Yarza de los Ríos (Comp.).¿ Quién es el sujeto de la discapacidad*, 155–181.

Chapter 4
Healing, Land, and Spirituality: Decolonizing Disability Through Traditional Practices

Abstract This chapter delves deeply into the core links among healing, land, and spirituality and considers their role as the primary factors in decolonizing disability in Latin America. It is developed on the basis of Indigenous knowledge systems from Abya Yala, it not only puts forward Western biomedical and neoliberal frameworks but also goes ahead and rejects them. It, however, points at a relational interpretation of disability as one brought about historically and politically through colonial violence, land dispossession, environmental injustice, and epistemic erasure. Indigenous healing methods such as curanderismo, shamanic plant medicine, Afro-descendant spiritual traditions, and community-based rituals are studied not just as cultural choices to Western medicine but as holistic systems of care that embrace the whole body, mind, spirit, community, and territory. These methods help to restore equilibrium by dealing with issues of spiritual disharmony, collective trauma, and broken ties with land and ancestors. The chapter also positions disability within a larger context of inequality and pointedly deals with issues such as forced migration, politically and economically motivated land grabbing, climate change, and pollution that the Indigenous and Afro-descendant people are exposed to and which contribute to health disparities among them. Community-centered healing models and disability justice movements are portrayed as resistance grounds that highlight collective care, cultural continuity, and participatory knowledge production. By emphasizing Indigenous practices, the chapter insists that the concept of epistemic justice is applied and health, disability, and care frameworks are fundamentally reoriented. It comes to the point that decolonizing disability means not only stopping with the incorporation of the marginalized within the colonial systems but also moving on to the non-violent Indigenization that recognizes land, spirituality, and relationality as the core of healing, justice, and collective liberation.

Keywords Disability · Decolonization · Indigenous healing · Spirituality and Latin America

S. M. Thomas and R. Veerabathiran, *Disability and Decolonial Thought in Latin America*, SpringerBriefs in Modern Perspectives on Disability Research,
https://doi.org/10.1007/978-981-95-8950-0_4

4.1 Introduction

The amalgamation of healing, land, and spirituality in Latin America poses a substantial epistemological dilemma to the application of Western biomedicine and the sociopolitical aspects that have always considered disability as a pathological condition. Being a radical change in perspective, it is rooted in decolonial praxis which not only dismantles but also redefines the very constructs of colonialism regarding normalcy, productivity, and embodiment by putting Indigenous worldviews at the forefront of the discussion, where disability is not seen as an individual shortcoming but a collective experience that has been influenced by historical trauma, environmental dispossession, and cultural continuity (Lapierre, 2023).

In Abya Yala—the name given by the Indigenous people to Latin America—prosperity is always considered to be holistic by the local communities, thus physical, spiritual, communal, and ecological dimensions are integrated into a unified concept of health that does not allow Fragmentation (Castro Romero et al., 2020). The use of traditional healing methods such as curanderismo, shamanic rituals, and community-based ceremonies is not restricted to the purposes of therapy but is also regarded as the means of resistance against the obliteration of Indigenous knowledge systems under colonial modernity in the first place (Schmidt, 2021; Tafur et al., 2009).

The ontological structure positions land, above all, as a major element. The Indigenous peoples in Latin America view their territories not simply as resources but as living beings with the attributes of past events, gods, and nature use. Their forced removals from the land of their ancestors—as a direct result of colonialism and the present-day exploitation of resources—disrupt the intergenerational passing of the healing knowledge and break the people-place bond, which is the cause of what some researchers call "suffering due to loss of territory." This type of spiritual disunion is expressed not only as psychical but also as bodily suffering, that is, it raises the rates of depression, suicidal thoughts, and chronic diseases in the displaced populations, especially in the youth, to a great extent (Hernández et al., 2024). On the other hand, the land-based rituals, farming, or pilgrimage become a healing process that not only reaffirms the indigenous peoples' rights over the land but also revives the languages, and brings back the worldviews where people and nature are in a reciprocity relationship.

The act of spirituality, in addition to mediating the healing process and being a source of resistance, played an important role in this manner. Various religious and spiritual ways of coping such as entrusting one's suffering to God (confiar en Dios), taking part in communal pláticas (dialogues), and narrating sacred stories, have been the prime factors for the mental health resilience of Latinx communities (Stege & Godinez, 2022). Such rites are usually the result of syncretic traditions that unite Catholicism with the spiritual practice of the Indigenous and African, thus developing hybrid systems of care that go beyond institutional religion (Abalos, 2006). However, spiritual frameworks do not draw a line between the personal and the political; instead, they see healing as something that is very much connected with justice, autonomy, and collective liberation (Comas-Díaz, 2024). The Chicano-Indigenous pedagogical models being one example, teaching can be a healing art when it affirms cultural identity, questions knowledge domination, and creates environments of hopeful resistance (Villanueva, 2013).

Disability cannot be viewed separately from the colonization, violence, and systemic alienation that have left their marks. Indigenous peoples suffer from very high rates of disability, the main cause of which are existing structural inequities and their intersections with culturally specific notions of embodiment and difference (Hernández-Wolfe, 2011). These inequities include poverty, lack of health care, and exposure to political violence. Most Indigenous peoples see disability not as a medical problem but rather as a different way of life, some even see it as closer to the spirit. In Indigenous cosmologies, diversity in body and mind is something that society needs for balance and is thus permeated with spiritual insight. So, in the case of decolonizing disability, rather than just mere inclusion, a radical change in the perception of who creates health knowledge, whose healing practices are approved and how land, language, and spirituality are acknowledged as main factors in wellness revival is absolutely necessary.

In this chapter, healing, land, and spirituality are represented as inseparable aspects which together serve to decolonize disability in Latin America and thus, pose a challenge to the biomedical, individualizing and productivity-centered paradigms. It presents the Indigenous ways of knowing as the very basis for allowing us to see disability as a condition that is not only relational but also historically defined and thus, shaped by colonial atrocities, the taking away of land, and the cultural struggle to survive rather than a mere biological defect. The Indigenous healing practices, land-based ceremonies, and spiritual worldviews are not seen as just the other options to Western medicine but as the extensive political and ethical interventions, which have the power to bring back the collective memory, the ecological justice, and the embodied dignity, among others. In this connection, the chapter claims that the decolonization of disability needs more than the reform of laws or the imparting of cultural sensitivity; what it really requires is the engagement of knowledge, power and care in the patterns of Indigenous understanding of the ´whole´ where justice, healing and liberation are not only interconnected but also established within the everlasting bonds of people, land, and spirit.

4.2 Spiritual Healing Practices: Key Differences in Latin America

Healing and wellness through indigenous lenses in Latin America manifest a striking contrast to Western biomedicine and its assumptions, namely, those of disability, health, and the body's, mind's, spirit's, and land's interrelation. Holistic models like these are based on what researchers' term Abya Yala—a native word for the Americas that denotes a viewpoint based on relationships, give-and-take, and harmony with the universe (Castro Romero et al., 2020).

Spiritual healing practices over the entire Latin America—almost one region with their different cultures, histories, and environments—are the result of a very complex fusion of the Indigenous, African, and European religions. These systems are thoroughly different from the Western biomedical ones in that they give priority to the holistic view which includes body, mind, spirit, and land as inseparable parts of health. So instead of treating disease as a mere physiological dysfunction, spiritual healing attempts to restore harmony in the relational, ancestral, and cosmological domains, or what scientists call "spiritual disharmonies" that are caused by the disconnection from oneself, the community, the land, and the sacred (Hernández et al., 2024). One of the most important differences among these practices is that they have different epistemological foundations, ritual forms, therapeutic goals, and social functions, which vary a great deal from one country, ethnicity, and region to another. Healing cannot thus be limited to the clinical intervention only; it has to include reconnection to the land, renewing the culture, restoring the language, and the solidarity of the community.

The idea of buen vivir (living well) is at the heart of the Indigenous models of well-being and it stands in stark contrast to the Western view of bienestar (well-being) which is mainly concerned with the individual's happiness or the physiological state being normal. Buen vivir is the product of the Andean and Amazonian worldviews that hold human thriving as being vitally dependent on maintaining the integrity of the ecosystem, passing down the ancestors' wisdom, and social consensus (Castro Romero et al., 2020). Human beings are viewed as part of the cosmos in such worldviews and the body is not an isolated biological entity but a node within a web that connects not only family and community but also nature spirits, sacred geography, and cosmological forces. So, in such interpretations, illness or disability is seen as a sign of an imbalance in these relationships—which could also be referred to as "spiritual disharmony" and not considered as a problem with the body functions. For example, the Emberá Dobida tribe in Colombia is affected by severe mental distress caused by a conflict that has displaced them. One of the symptoms of psychological distress during this period is an increase in youth suicide rates. Studies suggest that the problem is closely associated with the crying of the territory—the emotional, physical, and existential pain brought about by the loss of the connection with the ancestral land through forced separation (Hernández et al., 2024).

One major distinction can be seen in the classification of healers and their cosmological view. In Mexico, curanderismo is a syncretic system that combines the medicinal use of the Nahua with the Catholic symbolism and Spanish folk healing. Curanderos and curanderas (healers) frequently give names to certain diseases such as susto (fright sickness), mal de ojo (evil eye), or espanto (traumatic soul loss), and each of these diseases is treated with particular rituals that include herbs, prayers, eggs, candles, or even animal parts to restore the spiritual equilibrium (Tafur et al., 2009). Healing ceremonies can incorporate limpias (spiritual cleansings) with the help of fragrant plants or smoke, done, in parallel, with consejos—counseling dialogues that join emotional support and moral guidance. This approach gives a lot of importance to personal power, family reconciliation, and divine intervention by means of one being able to trust God ("trusting in God"), which faith is thus positioned not as a passive resignation but an active coping strategy that nurtures resilience among people who are going through mental distress or are disabled (Stege & Godinez, 2022). Figure 4.1 depicts the spiritual healing in Latin America and the different Western medicine approaches.

On the other hand, visionary plant medicine becomes the main focus in Amazonian shamanism among the Shipibo-Konibo in Peru or the Yanomami in Brazil, for instance. It takes the form of ayahuasca ceremonies guided by the shamans who are called vegetalistas. The shamans carry out these ceremonies involving psychoactive plant brews that bring about altered states of consciousness for the participants who then take to facing the spiritual beings, getting back their lost soul parts, and finding out the main cause of their suffering which is believed to be either through energetic intrusions or conflicts with ancestors 4. In this case, the healer does not perform the role of a counselor but rather acts as a mediator between the world of the living and that of the unseen, employing icaros (sacred songs) to traverse and negotiate healing with the plant spirits in the non-ordinary realities. This strategy points toward a belief system where disease is viewed as a spiritual assault or karmic imbalance and thus, the situation calls for direct interaction with the metaphysical powers rather than mere psychological self-exploration.

A different modality is that of spirit possession and ancestor veneration in Afro-descendant communities, especially in Brazil, where practices of Umbanda, Candomblé, and Quimbanda are mentioned. Healing is done in trance states where the mediums are taken over by the spirits who are leading the way—like pretos velhos (wise elder souls) or caboclos (Indigenous Forest spirits). These spirits guide, provide remedies, and offer emotional support (Schmidt, 2021). Afro-Brazilian traditions, unlike the individualistic nature of curanderismo or the personal intensity of shamanism, have a strong emphasis on community presence, rhythmic drumming, dancing, and other offerings to keep the cosmos in harmony. The disease is usually seen as a consequence of not respecting one's spiritual duties or not doing what one has come to this world for, thus making healing a process that has both medical and moral dimensions.

The main point of differentiation comes from the way the systems approach modernity and institutional power. Some of the traditional healers conduct their practice totally outside the state control while others have been assimilated into health care projects that are run by the govt. in a formal way, especially in the case of Ecuador and Bolivia where constitutional amendments got plural identities and Indigenous autonomy recognized. However, there are still barriers such as language issues, lack of cultural sensitivity in clinical areas, and the invisibility of non-Western methods in mainstream psychiatry (Hernández et al., 2024). One of the major issues of decolonization of mental health is the necessity to validate diverse healing paradigms and change the healthcare policy to where support of intercultural collaboration, land return, and epistemic justice as a start to well-being would be the main policy.

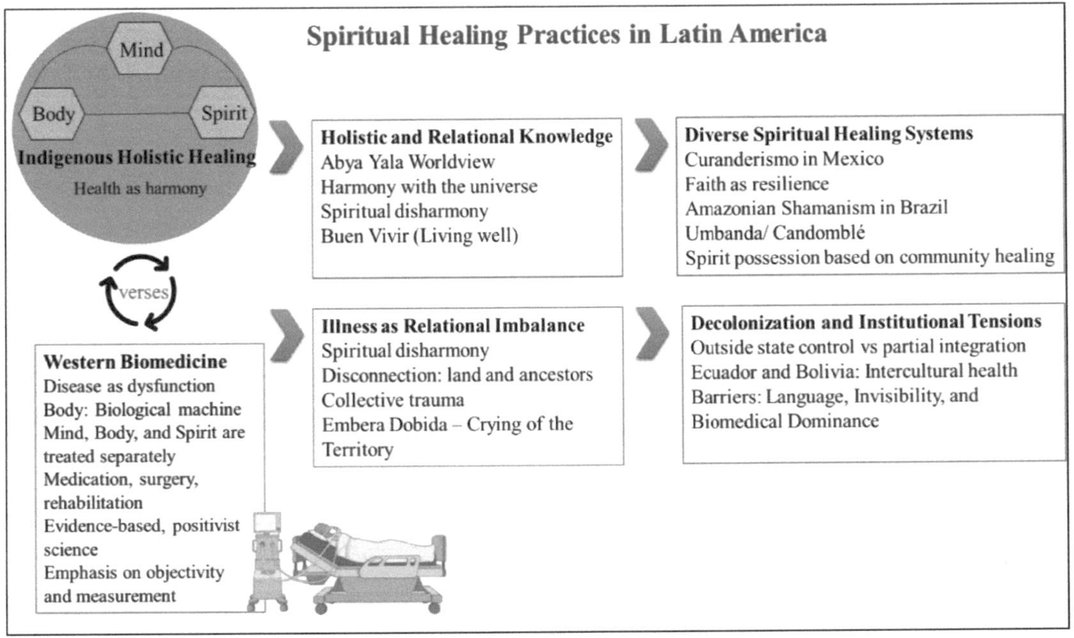

Fig. 4.1 Spiritual healing practices in Latin America. The figure contrasts Indigenous holistic healing worldviews with dominant biomedical approaches, highlighting relational understandings of health, illness, and decolonial tensions. This figure conceptualizes spiritual healing practices in Latin America through an Indigenous holistic lens and situates them in contrast to Western biomedicine. Indigenous holistic healing is represented as an integrated relationship between mind, body, and spirit, where health is understood as harmony within the self, community, nature, and the universe. Whereas Western biomedicine is grounded in a positivist and reductionist scientific paradigm that conceptualizes health and illness primarily through biological processes. It is based on empirical observation, laboratory diagnostics, and standardized clinical interventions, emphasizing objectivity, measurement, and reproducibility

4.3 Community-Centered Healing Practices and Collective Care

In Latin America, using community-centered healing practices and collective care for the disabled signifies a significant junction of disability justice, decolonial health approaches, and grassroots rehabilitation efforts. Primarily, these practices offer support among peers and include the use of traditional medicines while trying to alleviate both the social and health disparities (Fitzpatrick et al., 2024; Schmidt, 2021). The methods are unavoidable there since the disable population is not only limited in their rights to rehabilitation and integration into the community but also subjected to health inequalities, though the legal framework in some countries like Colombia has improved the situation a little (Toro-Hernández et al., 2019). The colonial past of the Global South has been very intertwined with disabled people and has significantly contributed to their isolation and thus the demand for decolonial perspectives in disability studies and practices has become needed (Meekosha, 2011).

The principles of disability justice, which frequently coincide with critical feminist inquiry, support and, moreover, argue for giving priority to the voices and viewpoints of the very outsiders, thereby mirroring the intersectional experiences of the disability communities (Goulden et al., 2023; Li et al., 2021; Tadman, 2023). This outline is of very much significance in Latin America, where the indigenous peoples, for instance, are perceiving disabilities in the light of their distinct worldviews and cultural practices, besides the disabling conditions forced by colonialism and poverty (Lapierre, 2023). The phrase "disability justice for collective liberation" declares war on ableism in every corner of the social structure, including education, public policy, and public places (Li et al., 2021).

Community-based inclusive development (CBID) interventions represent a critical aspect of rights projection for PWDs that are high in participation of communities in Latin America. These interventions are a direct answer to the existing gap of studies regarding the specific requirements of PWDs, which is the major cause of the deployment of improper programs. It is impossible to have a successful CBID without giving preference to the needs that have been prioritized and learning from communities in Latin America through sharing their experiences (Bachfischer et al., 2023). One of the reasons for this situation is that these programs usually coincide with community-research partnerships where the community members are the co-creators of knowledge, supporting the research process, and tackling the issues of health and lack of community participation (Suarez-Balcazar, 2020).

The Latin America region has seen a pronounced incline toward community-based and deinstitutionalized care models in terms of rehabilitation measures, especially when it comes to the treatment of persons with severe mental disorders. For example, Colombia, Costa Rica, and Peru are all making changes to their mental health systems so that they can be more supportive of the disabled community and even provide employment opportunities for them (Cubillos et al., 2020). Yet, some issues still exist, such as the fact that access to primary healthcare for adults with disabilities is very limited in most of the Latin American and Caribbean countries, a situation which is often exacerbated by the combination of systemic, economic, and cultural factors (Reichenberger et al., 2024). Research indicates that, in particular, Latinx immigrant families having children with disabilities view faith-based organizations and social services as the most important community resources for support, thus reflecting the important role of community networks in shared care (Suarez-Balcazar et al., 2022).

The notion of collective care is not limited to official healthcare systems; it also includes mutual assistance and companionship in communities. For instance, the engagement of the disabled activists in Latin America was practicing occupational therapy as reivindication of their rights from the traditionally oppressed area (Pino-Morán et al., 2023). This kind of activism has the support of feminists' critical views and highlights political acknowledgment and support as the major demands—though the Convention on the Rights of Persons with Disabilities gives them a push, its limitations in implementation are still a hindrance (Rebolledo-Sanhueza & Galaz-Valderrama, 2024).

Spiritual healing practices are very important in Latin America, they are often based on the indigenous peoples' traditional ways of life and the revival of Native American and African spiritualities (Espi Forcen, 2023; Schmidt, 2021). The practices which differ a lot between Mexico and Peru, for example, are already mixed up with religious doctrines and provide different or similar healing ways in the communities (Schmidt, 2021). This is a combination of a decolonial health approach that accepts and uses local knowledge systems, which have usually been disregarded by the Western medical models, as in (Meekosha, 2011; Schmidt, 2021). Community wellness worker models which have been implemented in different parts of the world among indigenous populations are becoming more and more recognized as a means to reduce healthcare access inequalities and facilitate holistic well-being. These models usually mix Indigenous and Western practices, stimulate community participation and take into account the local circumstances, thus creating supportive working conditions and giving priority to family-centered care (Fitzpatrick et al., 2024). Figure 4.2 depicts the role of a community wellness worker.

In Latin America, housing to PWDs accessibility is one of the major obstacles they have to overcome, even though it has been considered one of the main ways to support equal rights and independent living. Various sources claim that Brazil is responsible for the majority of the accessibility studies among PWDs in Latin America (Valderrama-Ulloa et al., 2023). Accessibility issues to urban public spaces in Latin American cities prevail even though there have been some legal and regulatory developments and assessments like street-level accessibility mapping are required to spot disparities (Orellana et al., 2020). It is possible to unravel barriers and facilitators to community participation for Latinx migrants with disabilities through the application of the social ecological model which shows the necessity of multi-level interventions (Suarez-Balcazar et al., 2020).

The COVID-19 pandemic has highlighted the weaknesses in the lives of disabled people and has put heavy reliance on the urgency of anti-violence advocacy grounded

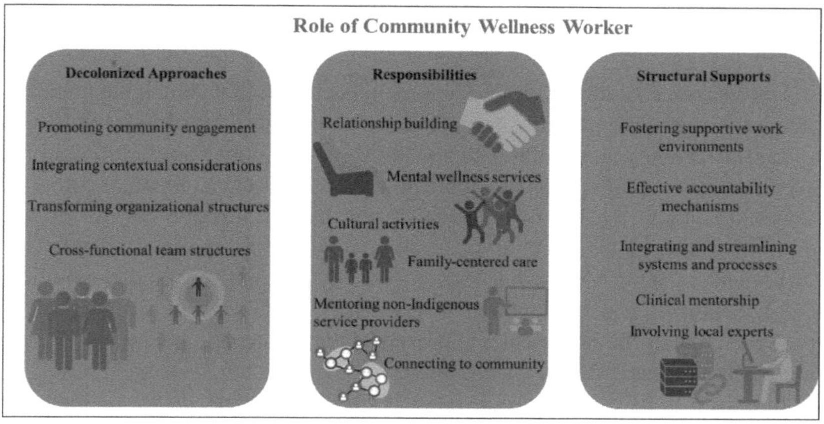

Fig. 4.2 Role of the Community Wellness Worker. The figure depicts the multidimensional role of community wellness workers through decolonized approaches, core responsibilities, and structural supports. The figure is organized into three thematic domains. The Decolonized Approaches emphasize community engagement, contextual and cultural integration, transformation of organizational structures, and cross-functional teamwork rooted in local knowledge systems. The Responsibilities of community wellness workers include relationship building, provision of mental wellness services, facilitation of cultural activities, delivery of family-centered care, mentoring non-Indigenous service providers, and strengthening connections between individuals, families, and the wider community. The Structural Supports highlight the systemic enablers necessary for effective practice, including supportive work environments, accountability mechanisms, streamlined systems and processes, clinical mentorship, and the active involvement of local experts. Collectively, the figure illustrates how individual practice, community engagement, and institutional support intersect to promote holistic and culturally responsive wellness care

in an intersectional disability justice framework (Shelton, 2021). The diverse government responses to COVID-19 in South America with respect to the disabled population revealed areas that have not been addressed well to cope with the unique risks that PWDs face when there is a crisis (Sakellariou et al., 2020). The foregoing incidents have made it all the more critical that policies and practices, which are disability-inclusive, be adopted worldwide and that such policies particularly include the disabled in disaster preparedness measures dealing with climate changes that affect the disabled disproportionately but still the stakeholders and decision-makers fail to include them (Engelman et al., 2022).

In Latin America, community-centered healing practices and collective care for disabled people are driven by community participation, cultural sensitivity, decolonial approaches, and the coexistence of traditional and modern health practices. The victory over the prevailing oppressive conditions, the right advocacy, and building of resilient communities that empower PWD and secure their full inclusion guaranteed through these efforts.

4.4 Disability: Colonial Violence and Land Dispossession

Latin America traces a very profound historical background in which the impairment is practically synonymous with colonial practices and injustices of a systemic nature. The disability studies, particularly those based in the Global South, are taking the Eurocentric views of things just the opposite way, by making it clear that colonialism has been an actor in the life of disabled people mainly through the use of forced assimilation, political violence, and economic exploitation (Connell, 2011; Grech, 2017; Lapierre, 2023; Meekosha, 2011). Out of the total disabled population of around 1 billion people worldwide, most of them (80%) are living in the Global South, which means the historical and present-day impacts are indeed very strong in these areas (Chouinard, 2014; Cleall, 2024).

Colonialism, in its various forms, has left a profound mark on the understanding and experience of disability in Latin America, often turning impairment into a direct or indirect consequence of violence and dispossession (Connell, 2011; Lapierre, 2023). An example of this is that the indigenous population of Latin America often sees and experiences disability through their own cultural lenses, which coexist with the disability reality created by colonialism, colonization, and forced assimilation. This situation is aggravated by the socio-economic, political, and cultural conditions under which the indigenous populations live, and which are the root causes of their higher disability rates (Lapierre, 2023). Historical violence in the form of displacement from and depriving of access to the native lands has been one of the chief causes of this, leading to a complete alteration of the social fabric, and rendering the access to health and other services increasingly difficult and unequal. For example, forced migration from the homeland (e.g., to Oklahoma) has rendered tribes physically and culturally isolated, and thus deprived of virtually all the resources necessary for a healthy community (mental health being among them). The geographical and infrastructural isolation of Indigenous people, especially in rural areas, combined with the meager services available directly aggravates their health problems and results in poor health among these communities (Maxwell & Thomas, 2023).

The land dispossession, which was a major aspect of colonialism, has left a deep historical memory that still impacts the Indigenous people of today, making them associate the loss of their territory with their suffering both physically and spiritually (Hernández et al., 2024; Lephakga, 2015; Mollett, 2021; Urrieta & Landeros, 2024). The study conducted among the Emberá Dobida community, which was forced to move because of violence, shows that the loss of their land results in very large emotional and health difficulties, such as feeling disconnected from others and not having enough food, which ultimately affects their ability to relate to others and the cultural ties with their mothers (Hernández et al., 2024; Maxwell & Thomas, 2023). The indigenous land tenure systems have been changing due to neoliberal policies aimed at privatization, and the increased vulnerability and dispossession of indigenous peoples have been the results (Levien & Upadhyay, 2022; Urrieta & Landeros, 2024). These situations are often connected with racialized gender violence and the extraction of natural resources, which further pushes women and girls with disabilities in indigenous communities into the margins (Acevedo et al., 2023; Aguirre, 2020; Altamirano-Jiménez, 2021).

In addition to this, the "medical model of disability" that perceives disabilities as mere instances to be cured has been a major paradigm since the 1800s; furthermore, it is particularly detrimental as it insists upon normalization. Besides, this theory frequently disregards the social and political factors that cause disability, such as the part that colonial violence plays (Zaks, 2024). To decolonize disability studies is to go through the process of critically questioning how Eurocentric thoughts have made disability experiences universal, thus isolating people in the Global South, and understanding that incapacity is very often due to the repercussions of colonial interventions, both past and present (Connell, 2011; Meekosha, 2011). The case of disabled Indigenous Australians, for instance, is very much connected to the European settlement's continuous impact and the demand for the decolonization of disability-related concepts and practices (King et al., 2014).

In scholarly circles, the phenomenon of ableism mixes with the colonial influence, thus forming the conditions under which disabled and sick academics, mostly of marginalized origin, suffer more intensely from the performance-based systems (Brown & Leigh, 2018). These structural problems are likewise apparent in the legal and medical professions. Victims of domestic violence who have a mental disability commonly do not receive the needed aid within the legal systems, which points to a general incapability to provide different needs (Douglas & Harpur, 2016). Likewise, the South Asian Muslim immigrant families with autistic children face the difficulties of trying to comprehend disability through different cultural lenses, professional dynamics across cultures, and the lack of suitable services (Jegatheesan et al., 2010).

Countries in Latin America show a variety of ways to define and comprehend disability in the context of social protection laws, and very often this leads to discrepancies between the suggested definitions and the real practices (Pinilla-Roncancio, 2015). Health research in the area, while dealing with problems such as goiter and cretinism, sometimes masks the inequities, neocolonialism, and war that are the main causes of these health issues (Vrana, 2023). The implementation of community-based inclusive development for disabled people in Latin America is considered a right but it also requires very active community involvement and a clear understanding of the needs of the community (Bachfischer et al., 2023). The role of Physical Medicine and Rehabilitation (PM&R) has increased in Latin America, but still, the majority of disabled people are women, the elderly, and ethnic minorities in poor countries (Schiappacasse et al., 2019).

The decolonization demand in different areas like mental health and health promotion works toward the destruction of the colonial health right's legacy that ultimately gives rise to health inequities (Chandanabhumma & Narasimhan, 2020; Sepúlveda Jara & Oyarce Pisani, 2020). In the case of Chile, the emerging models that support collective mental health and interculturality are often unsuccessful as they are still under the colonial power system (Sepúlveda Jara & Oyarce Pisani, 2020). Moreover, the decolonization approach emphasizes that the Indigenous knowledge systems in Africa, for example, have been defining and depicting disability in a negative light, thus, leading to the exclusion of the disabled people (Ndlovu, 2023). The term "coloniality" denotes to such power structures that still exist today as they are the remnants of colonial rule and they still affect disability in different ways 1. Thus, the power of 'coloniality' has continued to prevail and hence, ableism needs to be critically evaluated if it is still being used as a colonial instrument in the places such as Canada, where the Indigenous people are being viewed as unhealthy and the stories of 'inspiring disability' are being told to maintain the colonial impacts (Hutcheon & Lashewicz, 2020).

Disability in Latin America is an issue that goes beyond the medical field and the affected individuals, but rather it is deeply rooted in the history and the current circumstances of colonization, land dispossession, and systemic violence. To tackle the disabilities associated with these issues a decolonial approach is needed, and this should take into account the social, cultural, economic, and political factors that impact the lives of disabled people and particularly those of Indigenous origin in a connected way.

4.5 Environmental Injustice and the Production of Disablement

The Latin American indigenous peoples suffer the most from the impacts of toxic exposure, climate change, and destruction of nature, which together are the main causes of disabilities in these communities (Auerbach et al., 2025; Lapierre, 2023; Saravia, 2020). The reason for this increased vulnerability lies in a complicated mix of factors, including the long history of marginalization, the economic status of the community, and the fact that these people depend heavily on the environment for their food and culture (Lapierre, 2023; Laborde et al., 2014; Monterrubio Solís et al., 2023).

The toxic exposure has a very large share in causing disability in the Indigenous communities. Malnutrition, lack of perinatal care, and exposure to toxic agents are among the prominent factors in low-income and middle-income countries, thus possibly resulting in a higher incidence of intellectual disability in Latin America (Mercadante et al., 2009). Industrial development and urbanization have often been going on without proper environmental protection measures causing the contamination of air, water, and soil which, in turn, affects the health of children in the area (Laborde et al., 2014). One example is that children in the Indigenous communities of the Brazilian Amazon can face severe lifelong disabilities due to snakebite envenomation whose treatment with antivenom is not easily accessible for them compared to other groups (de Farias et al., 2023). Moreover, when people are exposed to environmental contaminants their chances of getting infectious diseases may actually go up. Toxoplasma gondii is an example of such a microbe in agro ecosystems where the Indigenous people of Brazil along with their animals and the environment get contaminated, which poses a One Health challenge whereby the environmental factors determine the health of living organisms (Doline et al., 2023). The combined impact of such exposures results in a high rate of health disparities that consist of different diseases, chronic ones in particular, and developmental problems, that can turn into disabilities (Garza & Abascal Miguel, 2025).

Climate change is one of the main contributors to the increase in these vulnerabilities. Latin America and the Caribbean have been classified as very susceptible regions to the impacts of climate change (Fernández et al., 2023; Rubin & Rossing, 2012), with further forecasts that the effects will be even more drastic (Oxford Analytica, 2018). For instance, Indigenous women facing poverty and discrimination are the first to be affected by climate change and their existence is threatened (Saravia, 2020). The MugClimate change has a huge economic cost, which mainly hits the already marginalized and economically disadvantaged, especially in the case of rural Indigenous folks, who are then, indirectly, seen through the lens of droughts in Chile hitting their income and labor market situations (Pérez-Silva et al., 2023). Changing climatic conditions may have a great impact on the occurrence of extreme weather events and that very thing could be a cause behind migration, lack of food, and people getting hurt with the latter leading to a rise in the number of handicapped people (Auerbach et al., 2025; Mercadante et al., 2009). Natural resources and biodiversity are the main reasons for the region's reliance on environment, and in turn, this reliance leads to the destruction of ecosystems, public health hazards, and local areas losing their economies (Ramírez-Cando et al., 2025). The older people in Los Angeles as well as in other Latin American cities who are already in a vulnerable situation, especially the ones living in areas prone to floods, are the most affected by climate change impacts (Chávez-Alvarado & Sánchez-González, 2016). Moreover, the mental health of people living in such conditions would be greatly affected by the combined effect of climate change, pollution, and diseases like COVID-19, thus, the burden of health continues to grow (Marazziti et al., 2021).

Ecological destruction, which is usually the case with the prevailing economic models and state policies, leads to the loss of land and resources to the native peoples, who are thus losing their means of production and social reproduction in the form of traditional food systems (Mercadante et al., 2009). Sharing their health, as well as being able to consume only poor-quality food, and suffering from long time weaknesses and other health problems that may turn into disability is part of their health and well-being issue that (Olmedo et al., 2020) also points to. Through the term "grieving geographies," Black and Indigenous women in Mexico are described as mourning not only the loss of lagoons to the government and neoliberal policies but also community, members and cultural heritage loss, which in turn affects their mental and physical health (Rodríguez Aguilera, 2022). Dams that cut off rivers' longitudinal connections, for example, have an adverse effect on fish species that are important for the local ecosystems and hence the Indigenous tribes that depend on them (Duarte et al., 2021). The prevalence of microplastics in nature is another pressing issue worldwide; although nothing is certain about their long-term effects on living and non-living resources, there is some proof at least that they are dangerous for the main species and can also lead to wider geographical destabilization (Sridharan et al., 2021).

The convergence of these elements brings about a syndemic scenario whereby, within the Indigenous populations, the health inequities and vulnerabilities are magnified (Granados et al., 2023). In Latin America, the Indigenous people are often marginalized, and the cultural differences constitute a barrier to the access of healthcare services, this was the case during the COVID-19 pandemic (Meneses-Navarro et al., 2020). The pandemic made the indigenous people even more vulnerable and besides that, their situation was made worse by remoteness and institutional racism. Yet, the Indigenous communities have a lot of resilience strategies, but the continuous extraction of resources and poor governmental support diminish their adaptability (Arsel & Pellegrini, 2022; Weber et al., 2021). Also, the absence of disability-inclusive climate change adaptation strategies aggravates the situation (Auerbach et al., 2025), and there is an urgent demand for research that applies intersectional and decolonizing methods to tackle the double discrimination of racism and disability (Daniels-Mayes, 2023). Among the Indigenous population, health disparities cover infectious diseases, malnutrition, and chronic conditions. All of these factors need to be looked at comprehensively in order to develop public health strategies that are just and fair (Garza & Abascal Miguel, 2025). To a large extent, the health of the indigenous people will be improved only if the underlying structural issues such as social exclusion, racism, and discrimination in the healthcare systems are dealt with (Babyar, 2019; Cerón et al., 2016). Maternal health disparity remains a less explored area that includes high maternal mortality rates and inadequate access to services, and isolation caused by systemic barriers makes it worse (Serván-Mori & Meneses-Navarro, 2025).

4.6 Decolonizing Disability Frameworks Through Indigenous Praxis

Decolonizing disability frameworks through Indigenous praxis in Latin America is undoubtedly an urgent and critical area of research, especially when considering the copious number of disabilities among the Indigenous population due to systemic racism and historical marginalization. Such a paradigm shift requires a complete divorce from those Western models of disability that consider non-normative bodies and minds as a pathology, and it must go the long way to be based in Indigenous worldviews, knowledge systems, and lived experiences (Daniels-Mayes, 2023; Lapierre, 2023). The theory that is being advanced through the decolonization of frameworks recognizes that the situation with disabilities in Indigenous communities is not only a matter of biology but is very much connected with the negative impacts of colonialism, forced assimilation, and persistent socio-economic disparities.

The difference between the Indigenous perspective on disability and the biomedical model is considerable. The latter perceives disability only through the lens of an individual impairment while the Maya, for example, view it as part of life through the whole person approach that takes into account soul, community, and earth's health.

Such integrated view of disability sees normality and ability as products of culture that may vary dramatically among the Indigenous peoples who may even support neurodiversity and variances in physical appearance through the lack of stigma that is so common in the West. In that regard, this cultural backdrop has to be taken together with the brutal reality of disabilities that were either caused or intensified by the colonization process of violence that included poverty, environmental destruction, and political persecution (Lapierre, 2023).

A decolonizing approach to disability in Latin America also directly deals with the widespread health problems of Indigenous peoples such as infectious diseases, malnutrition, and chronic conditions. Health inequalities in this case are not only reflected in health outcomes but are also seen as the consequence of systemic inequalities and long-term marginalization (Garza & Abascal Miguel, 2025). To illustrate, the climate change effects, like droughts, will increase the susceptibility of Indigenous people, and at the same time, this will impact their employment and reduce their income. Stress caused by the environment might eventually lead to the birth of new disabilities or aggravate the existing ones, thus making it even more urgent to deliver the interventions that are culturally sensitive and contextually appropriate (Pérez-Silva et al., 2023).

Moreover, the "accumulation by dispossession" theory omnipresent in history and current situations is indispensable for grasping the factors leading to the Indigenous peoples' disability. The current dominating economic theories and governments' policies are a common cause for the stealing, i.e., the loss, of the Indigenous peoples' lands, resources, and even food systems; thus, they directly cause the extinction of Indigenous peoples' means of production and social reproduction. The Saxons' and the Romans' conquest of the British Isles, for example, not only affected the health and well-being of the local inhabitants but might also have accidentally resulted in the appearance of certain diseases through malnutrition and other health-related issues, leading to the incapacity of the tribal folks 5. The construction of megadams for hydropower, for instance, results in the disintegration of river systems, which creates hurdles for the migratory or diadromous fish that are the lifeblood for the local biodiversity and the Indigenous peoples, and consequently, it results in the extinction of the traditional ways of living and food scarcity (Monterrubio Solís et al., 2023). The Decolonizing Disability Frameworks through Indigenous Praxis in Latin America is depicted in Table 4.1.

The creation of decolonized disability frameworks is reliant on research that is both informed and directed by the Indigenous peoples with disabilities, deeming their experiences and Indigenous perspectives as the topmost priority. This method of participatory and co-creative research not only assures the cultural appropriateness and relevance of the research questions and interventions but also encourages the challenging of the very existing power dynamics in knowledge production. The "BlakAbility" commentary, though primarily addressing the Australian Indigenous peoples, mirrors the global need for an intersectional and decoupling approach to research Indigenous people living with a disability, which is no less pertinent in the Latin American context. A such approach, moreover, must in a way or the other, force to the surface the dual discrimination of racism and disability, which ever so

Table 4.1 Decolonizing Disability Frameworks Through Indigenous Praxis in Latin America

Analytical dimension	Dominant western / Colonial disability framework	Indigenous Praxis–Based disability framework	Mechanisms producing disability	Implications for indigenous peoples with disabilities	Decolonial policy & Research implications
Ontological View of Disability	Disability as individual pathology or impairment	Disability as relational, holistic life condition	Biomedical reductionism	Pathologization of non-normative bodies and minds	Shift frameworks from impairment-focused to relational and cultural models
Knowledge System	Universalized Western medical epistemology	Indigenous worldviews, cosmologies, and lived experience	Epistemic exclusion of Indigenous knowledge	Cultural misinterpretation of disability	Center Indigenous epistemologies in disability research and policy
Mind–Body–Community Relationship	Mind–body separation	Integrated self (soul–body–community–land)	Fragmentation of care	Loss of culturally meaningful healing	Design health systems recognizing holistic well-being
Normality and Ability	Fixed norms of ability and productivity	Culturally contingent and diverse notions of ability	Imposition of Western norms	Reduced stigma toward neurodiversity in Indigenous contexts	Avoid universalized disability benchmarks
Colonial Violence and Disability	Colonial history treated as external factor	Colonialism central to disability production	Forced assimilation, poverty, persecution	Intergenerational trauma and impairment	Policies must address historical trauma as disability determinant
Health Inequalities	Seen as service delivery gaps	Result of long-term structural marginalization	Malnutrition, infectious and chronic diseases	Higher disability prevalence	Integrate disability policy with social justice and anti-poverty programs
Climate Change and Disability	Climate impacts treated as environmental issues	Climate stress as disability-generating force	Drought, food insecurity, stress	Emergence or worsening of disabilities	Climate adaptation strategies must include disability lens

(continued)

Table 4.1 (continued)

Analytical dimension	Dominant western / Colonial disability framework	Indigenous Praxis–Based disability framework	Mechanisms producing disability	Implications for indigenous peoples with disabilities	Decolonial policy & Research implications
Political Economy	Disability detached from economic systems	Disability linked to accumulation by dispossession	Land theft, resource extraction	Loss of livelihoods and social reproduction	Regulate extractivism; protect Indigenous land rights
Environmental Destruction	Environmental harm viewed separately	Environmental injustice central to disablement	Megadams, mining, biodiversity loss	Food scarcity and health decline	Environmental governance must include disability justice
Research Methodology	Expert-driven, extractive research	Participatory, co-creative Indigenous-led research	Knowledge power imbalances	Misrepresentation of Indigenous disability	Mandate Indigenous leadership in research design
Intersectionality	Disability addressed in isolation	Disability inseparable from race and coloniality	Dual discrimination (racism + ableism)	Compounded marginalization	Adopt intersectional disability justice frameworks
Health System Structure	Centralized, culturally insensitive	Community-based and culturally grounded	Institutional racism, peripherality	Barriers to care and support	Train health workers in Indigenous cultural competence
Indigenous Resilience	Often overlooked or romanticized	Active resistance and adaptive practices	Persistent extractive pressures	Strained coping mechanisms	Support Indigenous-led resilience initiatives
Core Principle of Decolonization	Inclusion within existing systems	Self-determination and cultural integrity	Colonial governance models	Limited agency of Indigenous peoples	Redesign disability policy around Indigenous sovereignty
Overall Framework Outcome	Medicalized, individualizing disability	Structural, relational, and justice-oriented disability	Colonial continuities	Persistent inequality vs dignified participation	Commit to decolonial disability justice as policy paradigm

often, the Indigenous peoples fall prey to in a most double manner (Daniels-Mayes, 2023).

In addition, the health systems in Latin America have been very often, and even the COVID-19 pandemic has shown it, institutionalized racism, cultural insensitivity, and lack of access among other things, the ones that have concerned. Peripherality and these systematic troubles work together in making the Indigenous peoples' access to basic healthcare and support services for disabilities. Nevertheless, the Indigenous groups continue to be very resistant, relying on diverse ways of dealing with the situation. On the other hand, their resilience is put to the test more and more and is sometimes even defeated by the persistent presence of mining activities and lack of adequate government support (Arsel & Pellegrini, 2022).

Decolonization of disability frameworks through Indigenous practices in Latin America requires a full understanding that integrates historical trauma, environmental injustice, socio-economic marginalization, and culturally specific interpretations of disability. It entails a dedication to Indigenous leadership in research and policy and the formulation of public health strategies that are not merely equitable but also based on the self-determination and cultural integrity of Indigenous peoples.

4.7 Conclusion

The reality of disability in Latin America, as shown in this chapter, cannot be explained in terms of Western biomedical or individualistic paradigms alone. Rather, it should be considered in the light of the historical and current realities of colonial violence, land dispossession, environmental degradation, and systemic inequality. The cosmologies of the Indigenous peoples of Abya Yala provide the world with radical perspectives that view disability in terms of relationships and community, as well as being bound to spiritual, ecological, and social aspects. Healers, in this way, are not only limited to the alteration of clinical interventions but include the restoration of balance between humans, land, ancestors, and the divine. The chapter, while emphasizing Indigenous and Afro-descendant healing practices, reveals that spirituality and land-based care act as resistance to the dominant epistemology and cultural erasure. The challenge to ableist presumptions of productivity and normalcy comes from these practices, which, in fact, acknowledge that bodily and mental diversity is an essential aspect of community rather than that which needs to be corrected. The models of community-based healing and collective care further act against the colonial hierarchy by placing belonging, sharing of knowledge, and culturally grounded approaches to disability justice at the core of the discussions. The chapter emphasized the partnership of environmental injustice and extractivist economies in deliberately making people disabled, especially among Indigenous communities whose existence and survival depend on their land. Therefore, recognizing disability means confronting those conditions that harm, viz. climate change, poison exposure, and compulsory migration. Decolonization of disability, in the end, requires not only reforms in policy or acknowledgment of cultures, but also the power of the Indigenous people in the areas of research, health care, and government. Making land, spirituality, and relationship the main focus is a prerequisite in the establishment of futures based on respect, healing, and liberation of the whole community.

References

Abalos, D. T. (2006). The personal, political, historical and sacred drama of transformation: Cultural implications for Latinos, Latinos with disabilities, and those who provide services and support. *Journal of Religion, Disability & Health, 9*(4), 29–54. https://doi.org/10.1300/J095v09n04_03

Acevedo, M. L., García, X. E., & Moctezuma, A. (2023). Violencias de género hacia mujeres y niñas indígenas con discapacidad en América Latina. *Cahiers franco-latino-américains d'études sur le handicap, 1*, 18. https://doi.org/10.56078/cfla_discapacidad.159

Aguirre, K. K. D. (2020). Colonized masculinities and femicide in Latin America. *Revista Crítica Histórica, 11*(22). https://doi.org/10.28998/rchv11n22.2020.0023

Altamirano-Jiménez, I. (2021). Indigenous women refusing the violence of resource extraction in Oaxaca. *AlterNative: An International Journal of Indigenous Peoples, 17*(2), 215–223. https://doi.org/10.1177/11771801211015316

Arsel, M., & Pellegrini, L. (2022). Indigenous people, extractive imperative and Covid-19 in the Amazon. In *COVID-19 and international development* (pp. 137–146). Springer International Publishing. https://doi.org/10.1007/978-3-030-82339-9_10

Auerbach, A. M., Abdukhalilov, A., Sacks, A., & Yusupov, D. (2025). Climate change and disability-inclusive adaptation: Qualitative evidence from Uzbekistan. *The Journal of Development Studies*, 1–18. https://doi.org/10.1080/00220388.2025.2530480

Babyar, J. (2019). In search of Pan-American indigenous health and harmony. *Globalization and Health, 15*(1), 16. https://doi.org/10.1186/s12992-019-0454-1

Bachfischer, A., Barbosa, M. C., Rojas, A. A. R., Bechler, R., Schwienhorst-Stich, E. M., Kasang, C., Simmenroth, A., & Parisi, S. (2023). Implementing community based inclusive development for people with disability in Latin America: A mixed methods perspective on prioritized needs and lessons learned. *International Journal for Equity in Health, 22*(1), 147. https://doi.org/10.1186/s12939-023-01966-8

Brown, N., & Leigh, J. (2018). Ableism in academia: Where are the disabled and ill academics? *Disability & Society, 33*(6), 985–989. https://doi.org/10.1080/09687599.2018.1455627

Castro Romero, M., Lorenzo Ruiz, A., & Melluish, S. (2020). Reimagining 'mental health' from the cosmovision of Abya Yala (Latin America). *International Review of Psychiatry, 32*(4), 299–302. https://doi.org/10.1080/09540261.2020.1782597

Cerón, A., Ruano, A. L., Sánchez, S., Chew, A. S., Díaz, D., Hernández, A., & Flores, W. (2016). Abuse and discrimination towards indigenous people in public health care facilities: Experiences from rural Guatemala. *International Journal for Equity in Health, 15*(1), 77. https://doi.org/10.1186/s12939-016-0367-z

Chandanabhumma, P. P., & Narasimhan, S. (2020). Towards health equity and social justice: An applied framework of decolonization in health promotion. *Health Promotion International, 35*(4), 831–840. https://doi.org/10.1093/heapro/daz053

Chávez-Alvarado, R., & Sánchez-González, D. (2016). Vulnerable aging in flooded households and adaptation to climate change in cities in Latin America: The case of Monterrey. *Papeles Poblacion, 22*, 9–42. https://doi.org/10.22185/24487147.2016.90.033

Chouinard, V. (2014). Precarious lives in the Global South: On being disabled in Guyana. *Antipode, 46*(2), 340–358. https://doi.org/10.1111/anti.12046

Cleall, E. (2024). Disability and postcolonialism. *Postcolonial Studies, 27*(1), 1–16. https://doi.org/10.1080/13688790.2024.2322252

Comas-Díaz, L. (2024). Decolonization: A personal manifesto. In *BIPOC and LGBTQ feminist radical visionaries* (pp. 21–36). Routledge. https://doi.org/10.1080/02703149.2022.2125617

Connell, R. (2011). Southern bodies and disability: Re-thinking concepts. *Third World Quarterly, 32*(8), 1369–1381. https://doi.org/10.1080/01436597.2011.614799

Cubillos, L., Muñoz, J., Caballero, J., Mendoza, M., Pulido, A., Carpio, K., Udutha, A. K., Botero, C., Borrero, E., Rodríguez, D., Cutipe, Y., & Torrey, W. C. (2020). Addressing severe mental illness rehabilitation in Colombia, Costa Rica, and Peru. *Psychiatric Services, 71*(4), 378–384. https://doi.org/10.1176/appi.ps.201900306

Daniels-Mayes, S. (2023). Researching Indigenous people living with a disability: The urgent need for an intersectional and decolonising approach (BlakAbility). *First Nations Health and Wellbeing-The Lowitja Journal, 1*, Article 100004. https://doi.org/10.1016/j.fnhli.2023.100004

de Farias, A. S., Cristino, J. S., da Costa Arévalo, M., Carneiro Junior, A., Gomes Filho, M. R., Ambrosio, S. A., Nickenig Vissoci, J., Wen, F. H., Azevedo Machado, V., Sachett, J., & Monteiro, W. (2023). Children growing up with severe disabilities as a result of snakebite envenomations in indigenous villages of the Brazilian Amazon: Three cases and narratives. *Toxins, 15*(6), 352. https://doi.org/10.3390/toxins15060352

Doline, F. R., Farinhas, J. H., Biondo, L. M., de Oliveira, P. R. F., Rodrigues, N. J. L., Patrício, K. P., Mota, R. A., Langoni, H., Pettan-Brewer, C., Giuffrida, R., Santarém, V. A., & Biondo, A. W. (2023). Toxoplasma gondii exposure in Brazilian indigenous populations, their dogs, environment, and healthcare professionals. *One Health, 16*, 100567. https://doi.org/10.1016/j.onehlt.2023.100567

Douglas, H., & Harpur, P. (2016). Intellectual disabilities, domestic violence and legal engagement. *Disability & Society, 31*(3), 305–321. https://doi.org/10.1080/09687599.2016.1167673

Duarte, G., Segurado, P., Haidvogl, G., Pont, D., Ferreira, M. T., & Branco, P. (2021). Damn those damn dams: Fluvial longitudinal connectivity impairment for European diadromous fish throughout the 20th century. *Science of the Total Environment, 761*, Article 143293. https://doi.org/10.1016/j.scitotenv.2020.143293

Engelman, A., Craig, L., & Iles, A. (2022). Global disability justice in climate disasters: Mobilizing people with disabilities as change agents: Analysis describes disability justice in climate emergencies and disasters, mobilizing people with disabilities as change agents. *Health Affairs, 41*(10), 1496–1504. https://doi.org/10.1377/hlthaff.2022.00474

Espi, F. (2023). From entheogens to evangelicalism: Spiritual practices among Hispanic/Latin Americans. *Psychiatric Annals, 53*(12), 545–549. https://doi.org/10.3928/00485713-20231109-01

Fernández, A., Franchini, M., Aragão, L., Carte, L., Pacheco, D., Ochoa Ochoa, L. M., Mohan, P. S., do Amaral Cunha, A. P. M., & Yglesias-González, M. (2023). Facing climate change across Latin America and the Caribbean. *Nature Climate Change, 13*(10), 1014–1019. https://doi.org/10.1038/s41558-023-01820-3

Fitzpatrick, K. M., Sjoblom, E., Puinean, G., Robson, H., Campbell, S. M., Fayant, B., & Montesanti, S. (2024). Examining global Indigenous community wellness worker models: A rapid review. *International Journal for Equity in Health, 23*(1), 90. https://doi.org/10.1186/s12939-024-02185-5

Garza, M., & Abascal Miguel, L. (2025). Health disparities among indigenous populations in Latin America: A scoping review. *International Journal for Equity in Health, 24*(1), 119. https://doi.org/10.1186/s12939-025-02495-2

Goulden, A., Kattari, S. K., Slayter, E. M., & Norris, S. E. (2023). 'Disability is an art. It's an ingenious way to live.': Integrating disability justice principles and critical feminisms in social work to promote inclusion and anti-ableism in professional Praxis. *Affilia, 38*(4), 732–741. https://doi.org/10.1177/08861099231188733

Granados, Y., Strozzi, A. G., Alvarez-Nemegyei, J., Quintana, R., Julian-Santiago, F., Santos, A. M., Guevara-Pacheco, S., Loyola-Sanchez, A., Goycochea-Robles, M. V., Juarez, V., Garza-Elizondo, M. A., & Pelaez-Ballestas, I. (2023). Inequity and vulnerability in Latin

American Indigenous and non-Indigenous populations with rheumatic diseases: A syndemic approach. *BMJ Open, 13*(3), e069246. https://doi.org/10.1136/bmjopen-2022-069246

Grech, S. (2017). Decolonising Eurocentric disability studies: Why colonialism matters in the disability and global South debate. In *Disability and colonialism* (pp. 6–21). Routledge. https://doi.org/10.1080/13504630.2014.995347

Hernández, F. A., Chamorro, J. M., & Pastas, N. M. (2024). Spiritual disharmonies among the emberá dobida: Territorial, bodily, and linguistic suffering. *Journal of Applied Youth Studies, 7*(1), 27–46. https://doi.org/10.1007/s43151-023-00111-0

Hernández-Wolfe, P. (2011). Decolonization and "mental" health: A Mestiza's journey in the borderlands. *Women & Therapy, 34*(3), 293–306. https://doi.org/10.1080/02703149.2011.580687

Hutcheon, E. J., & Lashewicz, B. (2020). Tracing and troubling continuities between ableism and colonialism in Canada. *Disability & Society, 35*(5), 695–714. https://doi.org/10.1080/09687599.2019.1647145

Jegatheesan, B., Fowler, S., & Miller, P. J. (2010). From symptom recognition to services: How South Asian Muslim immigrant families navigate autism. *Disability & Society, 25*(7), 797–811. https://doi.org/10.1080/09687599.2010.520894

King, J. A., Brough, M., & Knox, M. (2014). Negotiating disability and colonisation: The lived experience of Indigenous Australians with a disability. *Disability & Society, 29*(5), 738–750. https://doi.org/10.1080/09687599.2013.864257

Laborde, A., Tomasina, F., Bianchi, F., Bruné, M. N., Buka, I., Comba, P., Corra, L., Cori, L., Duffert, C. M., Harari, R., Iavarone, I., & Landrigan, P. J. (2014). Children's health in Latin America: The influence of environmental exposures. *Environmental Health Perspectives, 123*(3), 201. https://doi.org/10.1289/ehp.1408292

Lapierre, M. (2023). Disability and Latin American indigenous peoples. *Disability & Society, 38*(7), 1276–1280. https://doi.org/10.1080/09687599.2023.2192381

Lephakga, T. (2015). The history of the conquering of the being of Africans through land dispossession, epistemicide and proselytisation. *Studia Historiae Ecclesiasticae, 41*(2), 145–163. https://doi.org/10.17159/2412-4265/2015/300

Levien, M., & Upadhyay, S. (2022). Toward a political sociology of dispossession: Explaining opposition to capital projects in India. *Politics & Society, 50*(2), 279–310. https://doi.org/10.1177/00323292211016587

Li, L., Donato-Sapp, H. L., Erevelles, N., Torres, L. E., & Waitoller, F. (2021). A kitchen-table talk against ableism: Disability justice for collective liberation. *Equity & Excellence in Education, 54*(4), 361–374. https://doi.org/10.1080/10665684.2021.2047417

Marazziti, D., Cianconi, P., Mucci, F., Crowther, L. F., Chiarantini, I., & Della Vecchia, A. (2021). Climate change, environment pollution, COVID-19 pandemic and mental health. *Science of the Total Environment, 773*, Article 145182. https://doi.org/10.1016/j.scitotenv.2021.145182

Maxwell, D., & Thomas, J. (2023). Land allotment, transportation access, and indigenous maternal mental health. *Journal of Transport & Health, 33*, Article 101721. https://doi.org/10.1016/j.jth.2025.102203

Meekosha, H. (2011). Decolonising disability: Thinking and acting globally. *Disability & Society, 26*(6), 667–682. https://doi.org/10.1080/09687599.2011.602860

Meneses-Navarro, S., Freyermuth-Enciso, M. G., Pelcastre-Villafuerte, B. E., Campos-Navarro, R., Meléndez-Navarro, D. M., & Gómez-Flores-Ramos, L. (2020). The challenges facing indigenous communities in Latin America as they confront the COVID-19 pandemic. *International Journal for Equity in Health, 19*(1), 63. https://doi.org/10.1186/s12939-020-01178-4

Mercadante, M. T., Evans-Lacko, S., & Paula, C. S. (2009). Perspectives of intellectual disability in Latin American countries: Epidemiology, policy, and services for children and adults. *Current Opinion in Psychiatry, 22*(5), 469–474. https://doi.org/10.1097/YCO.0b013e32832eb8c6

Mollett, S. (2021). Hemispheric, relational, and intersectional political ecologies of race: Centring land-body entanglements in the Americas. *Antipode, 53*(3), 810–830. https://doi.org/10.1111/anti.12696

Monterrubio Solís, C., Barreau, A., & Ibarra, J. T. (2023). Narrating changes, recalling memory: Accumulation by dispossession in food systems of Indigenous communities at the extremes of Latin America. *Ecology & Society, 28*(1), 3. https://doi.org/10.5751/ES-13792-280103

Ndlovu, S. (2023). Indigenous knowledge systems in Africa: Exclusion of students with disabilities in South African higher education. *Curriculum Perspectives, 43*(Suppl), 127–140. https://doi.org/10.1007/s41297-023-00202-1

Olmedo, S., Valeggia, C., & Berra, S. (2020). Incipient neighborhood and socioeconomic stratification associated to nutritional status in Indigenous Qom preschoolers from Formosa, Argentina. *Ecology of Food and Nutrition, 59*(3), 279–293. https://doi.org/10.1080/03670244.2019.1700976

Orellana, D., Bustos, M. E., Marín-Palacios, M., Cabrera-Jara, N., & Hermida, M. A. (2020). Walk'n'roll: Mapping street-level accessibility for different mobility conditions in Cuenca, Ecuador. *Journal of Transport & Health, 16*, Article 100821. https://doi.org/10.1016/j.jth.2020.100821

Oxford Analytica. (2018). Climate change impacts will worsen in Latin America. *Emerald Expert Briefings*, (oxan-es). https://doi.org/10.1108/oxan-es239897

Pérez-Silva, R., Castillo, M., & Cazzuffi, C. (2023). Droughts and local labor markets. Studying heterogenous effects on women and indigenous people in Chile. *Economics of Disasters and Climate Change, 7*(2), 281–302. https://doi.org/10.1007/s41885-023-00130-4

Pinilla-Roncancio, M. (2015). Disability and social protection in Latin American countries. *Disability & Society, 30*(7), 1005–1020. https://doi.org/10.1080/09687599.2015.1059316

Pino-Morán, J. A., Zango-Martin, I., Rodríguez-Garrido, P., & Mora-Malo, E. (2023). Reivindicative occupational practices of activist with disabilities. *Cadernos Brasileiros de Terapia Ocupacional, 31*, Article e3510. https://doi.org/10.1590/2526-8910.ctoAO269135102

Ramírez-Cando, L. J., Alvarez, C. I., & Gualotuña, D. (2025). Overview based on latent dirichlet allocation: The case of study climate change research efforts in Latin America. *Environmental Monitoring and Assessment, 197*(7), 1–15. https://doi.org/10.1007/s10661-025-14291-0

Rebolledo-Sanhueza, J. A., & Galaz-Valderrama, C. (2024). Activismo y discapacidad en Latinoamérica: luchas por el reconocimiento. *Revista Estudos Feministas, 32*(1). https://doi.org/10.1590/1806-9584-2024v32n19076

Reichenberger, V., Corona, A. P., Ramos, V. D., Shakespeare, T., Hameed, S., Penn-Kekana, L., & Kuper, H. (2024). Access to primary healthcare services for adults with disabilities in Latin America and the Caribbean: A review and meta-synthesis of qualitative studies. *Disability and Rehabilitation, 46*(25), 6011–6020. https://doi.org/10.1080/09638288.2024.2320268

Rodríguez Aguilera, M. Y. (2022). Grieving geographies, mourning waters: Life, death, and environmental gendered racialized struggles in Mexico. *Feminist Anthropology, 3*(1), 28–43. https://doi.org/10.1002/fea2.12060

Rubin, O., & Rossing, T. (2012). National and local vulnerability to climate-related disasters in Latin America: The role of social asset-based adaptation. *Bulletin of Latin American Research, 31*(1), 19–35. https://doi.org/10.1111/j.1470-9856.2011.00607.x

Sakellariou, D., Malfitano, A. P. S., & Rotarou, E. S. (2020). Disability inclusiveness of government responses to COVID-19 in South America: A framework analysis study. *International Journal for Equity in Health, 19*(1), 131. https://doi.org/10.1186/s12939-020-01244-x

Saravia, P. F. (2020). Rocío SILVA SANTISTEBAN (ed.), Indigenous Women and Climate Change. *Diacronie. Studi di Storia Contemporanea*, (44, 4). https://doi.org/10.4000/12fgr

Schiappacasse, C., Guzmán, J. M., Dean, M. H., Corletto, S., Battistella, L. R., Imamura, M., Gutiérrez, J., Borelli, G., Muzio, D., & Micheo, W. (2019). Physical medicine and rehabilitation in Latin America: Development and current status. *Physical Medicine and Rehabilitation Clinics of North America, 30*(4), 749–755. https://doi.org/10.1016/j.pmr.2019.07.001

Schmidt, B. E. (2021). Spiritual healing in Latin America. In *The Routledge handbook of religion, medicine, and health* (pp. 113–125). Routledge. https://doi.org/10.4324/9781315207964

Sepúlveda Jara, R., & Oyarce, A. M. (2020). New and old knowledge aimed at decolonising mental health: Reflections and proposals from Chile. *International Review of Psychiatry, 32*(4), 334–339. https://doi.org/10.1080/09540261.2020.1767042

Serván-Mori, E., & Meneses-Navarro, S. (2025). Beyond disease burden: The urgent need to address maternal health disparities among Indigenous populations in Latin America. *International Journal for Equity in Health, 24*(1), 276. https://doi.org/10.1186/s12939-025-02600-5

Shelton, S. Z. (2021). Bringing the pandemic home: The shifting realities of intimate violence for disabled people in the time of COVID-19. *Disability Studies Quarterly, 41*(3). https://doi.org/10.18061/dsq.v41i3.8392

Sridharan, S., Kumar, M., Bolan, N. S., Singh, L., Kumar, S., Kumar, R., & You, S. (2021). Are microplastics destabilizing the global network of terrestrial and aquatic ecosystem services? *Environmental Research, 198*, Article 111243. https://doi.org/10.1016/j.envres.2021.111243

Stege, A. M. R., & Godinez, J. (2022). Trusting in God: Religious and spiritual support in mental health treatment expectations in Mexico. *Journal of Religion and Health, 61*(5), 3655–3676. https://doi.org/10.1007/s10943-022-01554-0

Suarez-Balcazar, Y. (2020). Meaningful engagement in research: Community residents as co-creators of knowledge. *American Journal of Community Psychology, 65*(3–4), 261–271. https://doi.org/10.1002/ajcp.12414

Suarez-Balcazar, Y., Early, A., Miranda, D. E., Marquez, H., Maldonado, A., & Garcia-Ramirez, M. (2022). Community-engaged asset mapping with Latinx immigrant families of youth with disabilities. *American Journal of Community Psychology, 70*(1–2), 89–101. https://doi.org/10.1002/ajcp.12578

Suarez-Balcazar, Y., Viquez, F., Miranda, D., & Early, A. R. (2020). Barriers to and facilitators of community participation among Latinx migrants with disabilities in the United States and Latinx migrant workers in Canada: An ecological analysis. *Journal of Community Psychology, 48*(8), 2773–2788. https://doi.org/10.1002/jcop.22452

Tadman, R. (2023). Who cares?: Ethics and practices of care and making change in contemporary queer performance production. *Contemporary Theatre Review, 33*(1–2), 61–79. https://doi.org/10.1080/10486801.2023.2173598

Tafur, M. M., Crowe, T. K., & Torres, E. (2009). A review of curanderismo and healing practices among Mexicans and Mexican Americans. *Occupational Therapy International, 16*(1), 82–88. https://doi.org/10.1002/oti.265

Toro-Hernández, M. L., Mondragón-Barrera, A., Múnera-Orozco, S., Villa-Torres, L., & Camelo-Castillo, W. (2019). Experiences with rehabilitation and impact on community participation among adults with physical disability in Colombia: Perspectives from stakeholders using a community-based research approach. *International Journal for Equity in Health, 18*(1), 18. https://doi.org/10.1186/s12939-019-0923-4

Urrieta, L., & Landeros, J. (2024). 'Until the land title is in my hands, the land is not sold!': Land, violence, and Indigenous survivance in Michoacán, Mexico. *Latin American and Caribbean Ethnic Studies, 19*(4), 459–478. https://doi.org/10.1080/17442222.2024.2353551

Valderrama-Ulloa, C., Ferrada, X., & Herrera, F. (2023). Breaking down barriers: Findings from a literature review on housing for people with disabilities in Latin America. *International Journal of Environmental Research and Public Health, 20*(6), 4972. https://doi.org/10.3390/ijerph20064972

Villanueva, S. T. (2013). Teaching as a healing craft: Decolonizing the classroom and creating spaces of hopeful resistance through Chicano-Indigenous pedagogical praxis. *The Urban Review, 45*(1), 23–40. https://doi.org/10.1007/s11256-012-0222-5

Vrana, H. (2023). Endemic Goiter and El Salvador's battle against cretinismo. *The American Historical Review, 128*(4), 1587–1617. https://doi.org/10.1093/ahr/rhad377

Weber, G., Cabras, I., Ometto, P., & Peredo, A. M. (2021). Direct management of COVID-19 at national and subnational level: The case of the western amazon countries. *Public Organization Review, 21*(4), 741–757. https://doi.org/10.1007/s11115-021-00565-x

Zaks, Z. (2024). Changing the medical model of disability to the normalization model of disability: Clarifying the past to create a new future direction. *Disability & Society, 39*(12), 3233–3260. https://doi.org/10.1080/09687599.2023.2255926

Chapter 5
Indigenous and Decolonial Disability Activisms

Abstract In this chapter, disability activism of Indigenous and decolonial backgrounds in Latin America is seen as a human-empowered and enlightened change of epochs and cultures that annul the holding on of disability to the Eurocentric worldview and the unfavorable perception of the differently-abled. By granting Euro-American culture a long-standing influence over the world, the author of this chapter supports their claim about the disability in Indigenous and Afro-descendant groups being irrevocably intertwined with colonialism, land theft, racial segregation, assimilation, and neoliberal rule. The chapter illustrates, through decolonial theory, Indigenous cosmology, feminist disability studies, and community psychology, the liberatory shift in disability activism in Latin America from mere inclusion to justice grounded in liberation. Directing the readers' attention to Indigenous-led movements, grassroots resistance among Black and rural communities, women- and youth-led initiatives, and transnational solidarity, the chapter emphasizes that activism is anchored in care of the community, cultural sovereignty, and self-determination. Attention is particularly directed toward protests, direct actions, and reclaiming public, territorial, and sacred spaces, as well as the increasing significance of digital activism in both visibility-building and alliance-making, notwithstanding the ongoing digital and language inequalities. Narratives, particularly through art, storytelling, oral histories, and embodied protests, were pointed out as necessary means to reclaim the power to narrate and to fight against the medicalization of disability and the provision of charity to disabled people as the only legitimate model of disability. The chapter also tackles criticisms of decolonial disability activism by emphasizing the necessity for, and sometimes the complexity of, negotiation with the international legal order, internal power differences, and co-optation by state and NGO structures. The chapter illustrates how the Indigenous and decolonial disability movements in Latin America are far from being merely rights-based struggles, but rather a complete and radical transformation of disability, justice, and community concepts that are based on Indigenous epistemologies and shared futures.

Keywords Disability · Decolonial activism · Digital disability · Disability movements · And disability resistance movements

S. M. Thomas and R. Veerabathiran, *Disability and Decolonial Thought in Latin America*, SpringerBriefs in Modern Perspectives on Disability Research,
https://doi.org/10.1007/978-981-95-8950-0_5

5.1 Introduction

In Latin America, indigenous and decolonial disability activism means reaching the most critical and transformative ways of understanding and dealing with disability, respectively. At the very core of their approach, they are the strongest challengers of the Eurocentric paradigms and have the capacity to properly integrate indigenous epistemologies and cultural practices (Ferrari, 2020; Lapierre, 2023; Roy, 2024). Therefore, this movement comes from the continent where disability is still produced or, at least, intensified by the process of and even the historical and ongoing colonialism, colonization, and forced assimilation into often very restrictive state structures (Lapierre, 2023; Ortega, 2023). These types of activism focus on community, cultural identity, and the unmaking of systemic oppression imposed by colonialism, which became a part of our history and is still present in different ways (Moura et al., 2024; Rodríguez & Inturias, 2018).

The classic way of looking at disability, heavily influenced by Western views, has made the very concept of disability European, thereby overshadowing the experiences and understandings of disability in the Global South, especially among the indigenous population (Grech, 2017; Meekosha, 2011; Roy, 2024). Among the challenges faced by decolonial disability studies, one is to correct this skewed viewpoint and, in doing so, to uncover the linkages between colonialism, disability, and social injustice, to examine the impacts of coloniality, and to suggest a new definition of disability that is culturally and contextually appropriate (Ferrari, 2020; Moura et al., 2024; Ortega, 2023; Roy, 2024).

In Latin America, indigenous peoples are not only living with their disabilities as a matter of their own worldviews and cultural practices, but they are also experiencing them through the lens of the colonial legacies. The legacies comprise the process of dehumanization of natives and the application of the violence of the ableist as a colonial means, with the logic of purification or elimination of the perceived defects. The socio-economic conditions that the indigenous peoples endure, along with the political violence, add up to the oppression and thus the disability in the native communities, acquiring its special characteristics (Hutcheon & Lashewicz, 2020; Lapierre, 2023).

Decolonial disability activism emerging in Latin America has been marked by its prevailing concern with confronting these power relations and seeking self-determination. For instance, among the mobilized means is the activist art which operates at the junctions of disability, non-normativity, and indigeneity, thus facilitating the decolonization and indigenization of the conceptualization of disability (Rice et al., 2021). This strategy takes into account that the fight for disability rights is really a part of the larger decolonial battles and cannot be detached from the historical oppression and marginalization periods (Daniels-Mayes, 2023). The activists also condemned the 'white-elitist veganism of the Global North' for being very restricted in its approach to the Latin American region by not taking into account its territorial, cultural, and economic specificities, thereby portraying the dominant advocacy models as neocolonial and universalizing (León, 2024).

Latin American activists with disabilities, particularly those in Chile, have practiced claiming occupations from their historically marginalized places by using methods such as deep interviews, group chats, and analyzing social media content to formulate their demands and to dispute the dominant narratives (Pino-Morán et al., 2022, 2023). The above-mentioned movements are not the only ones, as groupings have also sprung up in the form of counter-hegemonic sociopolitical discourses that recognize the experiences and views of the so-called disabled (Pino-Morán et al., 2022).

The larger framework of activism in Latin America, comprising the movements against neoliberalism and women's rights, among others, offers ample opportunity for these decolonial disability challenges (Shekha, 2011; Strawn, 2009). Researchers have increasingly acknowledged that an intersectional and decolonizing approach is the only workable one among the disabled indigenous peoples, one that is experienced and guided by those with the lived experience (Daniels-Mayes, 2023). This is the process of unlearning traditional Western academic practices and values that have been the oppressors of indigenous peoples throughout history (Gilroy et al., 2018).

The idea of "coloniality of ability" is presented as a concept of decolonial feminist theories, which aims at a critical examination of the definitions and ideas of disability in the Latin American context (Ferrari, 2020). Through the coloniality of ability concept, it is easier to see how disability was manipulated by the colonizers as an instrument to claim dominance over certain human beings and how, in the end, the concept actually expanded to include non-normal human beings and even native people (Ortega, 2023).

Moreover, the role of indigenous populations in the Community Psychology movement in Latin America can be seen, among other things, through the notion of participatory processes and community mobilization, as a decolonial action. The mentioned point of view intends to uncover the consequences of colonialism and to bring back the indigenous foundations that have been denied historically (Moura et al., 2024).

The significance of indigenous authority and guidance in disability research is underlined too, especially in areas like Australia, where new research methodologies are being created to align with indigenous people's values and daily life, and to take into account the past effects of racism and colonization that people had to endure (Gilroy et al., 2018; Hollinsworth, 2013; King et al., 2014; Puszka et al., 2022). One of the aspects taken into account in such a process is that Aboriginal people who are disabled usually face both racism and discrimination on the grounds of their disability, which is a critical and yet hugely neglected intersection that has been grossly underscored (Daniels-Mayes, 2023). Native viewpoints frequently disengage from the Western disability paradigms and claim the same position as to the conceptualization of the colonization resistance (Velarde, 2018).

In Latin America, both indigenous and decolonial disability movements are not just confronting but rather overturning the Eurocentric concepts of disability, bringing in the indigenous wisdom through cultural practices, and breaking down the colonial frameworks that have long created and kept the inequalities related to disability. The situation that is not only about promoting rights is also about a disruptive characterization of disability from the decoupling point of view, putting the community and self-determination at the forefront. The activists advocate for the "nothing about us without us" rule by ensuring that the decisions that impact disabled indigenous people's lives are taken in their company (da Nóbrega Rogoski et al., 2024; Daniels-Mayes, 2023; Ferrari, 2020; Lapierre, 2023; Moura et al., 2024; Ortega, 2023; Roy, 2024).

This chapter makes use of these foundational concepts to study Indigenous and decolonizing disability rights movements in Latin America through various interconnected facets. It begins by scrutinizing the impact of coloniality, ableism, and governmental authority on the situation in which disability activism arises, especially in the case of Indigenous and poor communities. After that, it goes on to give examples of resistance movements and organizations that disabled Indigenous activists have to face and negotiate within the community, culture, and political fight. Besides signaling the importance of art, storytelling, oral histories, and protest, the chapter views these means as tools for reclaiming agency, visibility, and narrative authority. The chapter then goes on to examine the tensions, potentials, and the future of decolonial disability activism, indicating how these movements reinterpret disability justice through the lenses of Indigenous knowledge, collective care, and self-determination in the Latin American context.

5.2 From Inclusion to Liberation: Decolonial Disability Justice

The convergence of coloniality, ableism, and the politics of resistance, especially in the decolonial disability justice movement in Latin America, displays the enormity of power structures that are historical and present, which systematically marginalize and exclude persons with disabilities (Ferrari, 2020; Lapierre, 2023; Meekosha, 2011). Coloniality, in the way Aníbal Quijano first presented it and subsequently, the way Walter Mignolo and others have continued to develop it, is a term for the unbroken power signatures of colonialism that conquered all erstwhile colonial territories, and afterward continued to influence knowledge, power, and even existence (Gandarilla Salgado et al., 2021; Mendoza, 2015; Salvatore, 2010). With this viewpoint, it becomes easier to see how the very concept of disability was born out of the colonial matrix, and this resulted in the emergence of ableist attitudes and practices that are tightly woven into the fabric of everyday life, institutions, and sometimes even academic disciplines (Hutcheon & Lashewicz, 2020; Meekosha, 2011; Roy, 2024).

Ableism has become one of the factors that developed through colonialism—discrimination and social prejudice against people with disabilities based on the assumption that the typical human abilities are superior, yet it is not a standalone phenomenon, but rather is very much connected to the colonial legacies (Hutcheon & Lashewicz, 2014, 2020). In the case of Latin America, the colonization process was very much disabling and tormenting for the native inhabitants, and the production of disabled people continues to be the case due to colonial-related events (Lapierre, 2023; Meekosha, 2011). For instance, during colonization, the imposition of Eurocentric notions of the "normal" body and mind resulted in the death and isolation of indigenous bodies and ways of knowing, which are still powerful and fragile forms of ableism—subtle and overt—today (Capella Palacios & Jadhav, 2020; Hutcheon & Lashewicz, 2020; Lapierre, 2023). The social and institutional institutions of education, health care, and social policies that have been in existence for a long time are evidence of this—they often overlook and ignore the individual needs of disabled persons and, instead, further the promotion of a single able-bodied ideal (Arroyo-Rojas, 2024; Gibson, 2012; Leal & Torres, 2024). The colonial power, which is one of the main ideas in decolonial thinking, has disability as a factor to control and classify the subjects, especially in the areas of Latin America in the colonial period (Gandarilla Salgado et al., 2021; Ortega, 2023).

The decolonial disability justice approach to politics of resistance against these intertwined systems of oppression is called for (Ferrari, 2020; Horta et al., 2023). This approach does not merely include but rather a considerable transformation of society and knowledge systems (Berthelot-Raffard, 2024; Jantzen, 2015). Decolonial disability justice in Latin America refers to the indigenous worldviews, such as "Bien Vivir," whose social life perspectives are opposite to the coloniality of power and assert collective well-being instead of individualistic, Western-centric concepts of productivity and ability (Quijano, 2016; Yellowhorse, 2022). This means not only that one must acknowledge but also that one must respect the different beings and knowings that have been buried by colonial and ableist narratives (Kallio-Tavin & Wexler, 2022; Lapierre, 2023).

One of the most significant pieces of the resistance puzzle is the very decolonization of disability studies. Disability studies have always had a strong European bias, which has been one of the main points of critique against them. They have been viewed mainly as Western concepts of disability extended universally while completely disregarding the cultural, historical, and geopolitical contexts of the Global South (Grech, 2017; Meekosha, 2011; Roy, 2024). A decolonial viewpoint argues that this epistemic dominance is challenged through the voices and epistemologies of the marginalized communities being accepted, mainly disabled academics and indigenous peoples, thus making the knowledge produced authentic and liberating (Lapierre, 2023; Roy, 2024; Vaughan et al., 2019; Woods et al., 2018). For example, critical autism studies stress the importance of autistic-led scholarship to maintain epistemological integrity and to ensure that the portrayal of autistic culture and the neurodiversity movement is accurate (Woods et al., 2018).

In addition, decolonial disability justice calls for a complete overhaul of institutional frameworks, primarily in the case of universities. North American universities, which give a lot of lip service to equity, diversity, and inclusion (EDI) promotion, are often blind to the needs of disabled people when it comes to accessibility, thus revealing an underlying "capitalism" that favors certain kinds of intellectual output (Berthelot-Raffard, 2024; Waterfield et al., 2018). In Latin America, the colonial narratives have been the leading force in shaping the universities, and the decolonization of the curriculum and teaching methods is the only way to eliminate the ableist practices and promote the creation of a more welcoming academic environment (Valenzuela, 2023). Acknowledging how coloniality influences the training of professionals, such as psychologists, in Latin America is part of this process, where often Western-centric models are reproduced that do not take into account local realities and indigenous healing practices (Capella Palacios & Jadhav, 2020; Sepúlveda Jara & Oyarce Pisani, 2020).

The fight against coloniality and ableism also includes certain areas, such as physical education, where not only the past but particularly in countries like Chile, the Whites and the able-bodied people have been the primary focus in the curriculum and pedagogical practices that have excluded the needs of disabled students (Arroyo-Rojas, 2024). In the same way, colonial ideologies are still active in the government policies, educational methods, and churches in Indonesia, where ableism is further supported (Setio, 2025).

The decolonial feminist methods are still deeply related to the comprehension and overcoming of the coloniality of disability. The feminisms of Latin America, which are decolonial in nature, scrutinize the relationship between gender and disability by the coloniality and at the same time, to a degree, they lead to the questioning of the dominant feminisms that mostly ignore the struggles of women with disabilities who are marginalized (de Lima Costa, 2020; Ferrari, 2020; Lyra, 2023; Mendoza, 2015). One example of this can be found in the work dealing with mothers, disabilities, and rurality in Chile, where it is pointed out that the so-called "modern/colonial/Western/urban" understandings of the subject matter are at times totally devoid of the context and therefore need decolonizing practices and knowledge (Rodríguez-Garrido & Pino-Morán, 2023). The interrelation of race, gender, and disability is very important in the process of undoing both colonialism and ableism in the field of research, especially when it comes to the issue of racial justice (Boda et al., 2022; Horta et al., 2023).

In Latin America, decolonial disability justice is a complex issue since it points out the colonialism and ableism in the past and present that have had negative influences on disabled individuals and communities (Ferrari, 2020; Lapierre, 2023; Ortega, 2023). It urges a radical re-structuring of society, production of knowledge, and political action to obtain liberation and equal rights that are real, not just the coming together of different parts (Berthelot-Raffard, 2024; Jantzen, 2015; Rodríguez & Inturias, 2018). Decolonial disability justice will be achieved by giving priority to oppressed voices, bringing back indigenous ways of knowing, and fighting against the coloniality of power that has come to the stream of us in all its forms (Kallio-Tavin & Wexler, 2022; Lapierre, 2023; Quijano, 2016).

5.3 Indigenous Disability Activism in Latin America

The emergence of the Indigenous-led disability movements in Latin America indicates a significant and very positive change from the typical, mostly externally imposed, models of disability advocacy toward the culturally appropriate and self-determined modalities. In the past, disability in Latin America was considered and dealt with through the lens of Western civilization, which almost always neglected to take into consideration the indigenous worldviews and the cultural practices coping with disability. The colonial period greatly influenced the perception of disability, which, in many cases, was through the lenses of pathology applied to the indigenous bodies and their existence, thus making it a reality where the concept of disability is inseparably linked with the colonial legacies and socio-economic conditions (Lapierre, 2023; Meekosha, 2011; Ortega, 2023).

Indigenous-led disability movements are marked by community-based organizing, which is in stark contrast to most NGO-driven models where such community-based organizing might unintentionally sustain colonial dynamics (Lapierre, 2023). Although NGOs are often the leading providers of essential services, sometimes their methods can be all-encompassing, and therefore, they end up casting aside the distinct experiences of indigenous people in the Global South (Meekosha, 2011). Instead, community-based projects are based on local knowledge and are carried out through collective action, where self-determination and the incorporation of indigenous beliefs in dealing with disability are highlighted. This local organizing detects that disability within indigenous communities is very much connected with the oppression of colonization, forced assimilation, and political violence that continue to this day. These movements create new ways of dealing with the colonial ontologies of disability by acknowledging non-normative bodies and identities through concepts from indigenous languages, such as "imbunches and ch'uqtas," which are used to describe the identities and experiences of people with disabilities in particular indigenous communities (Lapierre, 2023; Ortega, 2023).

The intersectionality of indigeneity, disability, land, and sovereignty is very central to these movements. For indigenous people, the land wasn't just a source of income but a very significant part of their religion and culture, symbolizing their ancestors, heritage, and identity (Yellowhorse, 2022). Colonizing nations have always treated the indigenous people in such a way that they took over their lands and made it impossible for them to live off it, consequently displacing them in terms of culture, and making it difficult for the community to support them; all these factors having a negative impact on the health and leading to disability creation (Lapierre, 2023; Yellowhorse, 2022). The struggle against colonialism, therefore, involves the defense of lands and territories, as they are places where not only the indigenous communities, but also the disabled members, can get their survival and self-determination (Yellowhorse, 2022). Thus, the term sovereignty goes beyond just political control to cover cultural sovereignty, which gives the indigenous community power to determine and deal with disability issues according to their own notions and practices that might be completely different from those imposed by outside, often ableist, definitions (Lapierre, 2023; Yellowhorse, 2022). This decolonial approach takes on the "coloniality of capacity," which refers to the myth that specific capabilities are always better than the rest, a concept that is very much a part of the colonial mindset (Ferrari, 2020).

Decolonial disability justice is a movement in Latin America that aims to eliminate and replace the existing colonial attitudes on disability (Ferrari, 2020; Meekosha, 2011). Among these is the rethinking of the research, especially in the disability studies discipline, which has been chiefly influenced by the Global North and has therefore disregarded the vast array of knowledge and the experiences of the native people (Meekosha, 2011). Activists are working for the decolonization of knowledge, and they are proposing methods and frameworks that are compatible with the indigenous ways of knowing and that also provide solutions relevant to the local context (Rodríguez & Inturias, 2018; Rodríguez-Garrido & Pino-Morán, 2023). It is a matter of ethics and politics to admit the presence of non-normative bodies and to make it possible for different bodies to live with respect and freedom (Ortega, 2023).

The sociodemographic factors and political violence that were largely by-products of colonial and neocolonial frameworks negatively impacted indigenous people's health and welfare the most (Lapierre, 2023). Consequently, the resistance movements are rallying behind the cause of disability rights along with the fights for environmental justice, land rights, and self-governance (Rodríguez & Inturias, 2018). These movements are revealing the way that the world responds to crises, for example, the COVID-19 pandemic, can draw out settler-colonial histories and capitalism, thus further isolating the indigenous people with disabilities (Yellowhorse, 2022). In the final analysis, the indigenous disability activism in Latin America is a revolutionary force, not only for the oppressed but also for the whole society, as it demands the very transformation of the existing societal structures and the recognition of the intrinsic worth and the sovereignty of the indigenous disabled lives (Lapierre, 2023; Ortega, 2023).

5.4 Case Studies of Resistance Movements and Organizations in Latin America

In Latin America, the various forms of mobilization that are frequented by the resistance movements and organizations focused on the rights of disabled people have also been connected to the movements led by indigenous people, Afro-descendants, feminists, and youth. Momentum built by transnational support is also a contributing factor in this intersectionality. The movements oppose the discriminatory practices against people with disabilities that have been a part of the region's history and are a result of socio-economic inequalities, which affect people with disabilities the most (Lapierre, 2023; Meekosha, 2011; Rebolledo-Sanhueza & Galaz-Valderrama, 2024).

5.4.1 Indigenous Disability Collectives in Mexico, Bolivia, and Colombia

Indigenous peoples in Latin America generally see disability through a different cultural perspective, which can sometimes result in the availability of protective traditional healing practices and, at the same time, the suffering of the disabled by the compounded marginalization that has been caused by colonization, forced assimilation, and political violence (Lapierre, 2023). It has been found that indigenous people with disabilities have to endure double- sided discrimination when accessing healthcare facilities, which comes from the combination of their indigenous identity with that of being disabled (Rivas Velarde, 2018). In Mexico, for example, there have been cases where studies have probed the requirements and the means of indigenous communities with disabilities in the likes of Oaxaca, showcasing their points of view through participatory research methods (Marshall et al., 2004). Such groups are often vocal about their lack of connection with the Western understanding of disability; instead, they want to consider disability in the context of their traditional worldviews and communal practices (Velarde, 2018).

Indigenous movements in Bolivia and Colombia have been a stronghold throughout history, advocating for group rights and self-rule (Schilling-Vacaflor & Flemmer, 2020; Van Cott, 2005). Besides land, culture, and politics, the disability issue is coming up as a quiet advocate within these movements. The plight of the indigenous peoples with disabilities is aggravated by their socio-economic circumstances, which are characterized by very high poverty levels (Campos, 2021). The disability activists in the indigenous areas are often the ones to speak out to the authorities, demanding more acknowledgment and power, particularly inspired by the international treaties, including the Convention on the Rights of Persons with Disabilities (CRPD) (Rebolledo-Sanhueza & Galaz-Valderrama, 2024). Still, the realization of these rights is a complex issue (Pinilla-Roncancio & Rodríguez Caicedo, 2022). These groups have both traditional and modern means of protest at their disposal, for example, in Bolivia, where disability activists have been demonstrating for government support, and in Chile against the Telethon's credibility (Brégain et al., 2022).

5.4.2 Grassroots Mobilization Among Afro-Descendant and Rural Communities

Moreover, Afro-descendant populations in Latin America are virtually non-existent in the social scene, as they suffer from racial discrimination, and, therefore, the significantly higher numbers of impoverished people are among them (Agudelo, 2010; Campos, 2021). The collective actions of these people are a result of their historical background of struggles for rights, land ownership, and cultural recognition that have led to some government policies like the anti-racial discrimination rights and affirmative action (Hooker, 2008; Paschel & Sawyer, 2008). Alongside these main movements, grassroots resistance actions for the disabled are growing but remain mostly hidden. For example, the Afro-indigenous and Indigenous-Kriol communities on the Caribbean Coast of Nicaragua are fighting for their right to self-governance against land invasion, which brings to the forefront the intricate relationship between ethnic identity, land rights, and possible disability repercussions due to conflict or environmental degradation (Montiel Valle, 2021).

The "maroon socioterritorial movements," which originated from runaway slaves, are still, to this day, excellent examples of social movements that aim to achieve political goals by using space as their main battleground. The geopolitical aspect of these movements has, in fact, been quite neglected by researchers who mainly look at peasant and indigenous movements in Latin America (Guillen, 2022). The movements, which are people-led at the root level, reveal their resistance through the territorial and functional transformation, and thus may inspire the creation of non-violent resistance scenarios that are Disability-friendly. The use of social media has been a significant factor in these communities' collective power, and it has also made new avenues for civic participation and advocacy available, although the issue of accessibility continues to be an essential and critical one, especially when it comes to disaster communications (Kent & Ellis, 2015; Lupien, 2020).

5.4.3 Women- and Youth-Led Disability Resistance Initiatives in Latin America

In Latin America, women with disabilities go through many forms of discrimination as they suffer from ableism, they are subjected to intolerance as women, and they are often very likely to become victims of violence and abuse, including domestic violence (MacKeigan, 2021; Pestka & Wendt, 2014). To this issue, women-led disability resistance movements become the prime means for the intersectional oppressions to be tackled. The "feminization of resistance" is an evident phenomenon in the case of Argentina's #NiUnaMenos (NUM), which is a significant transnational feminist mobilization aimed at eradicating gender-based violence and has already given birth to distinctive protest performances (Medina, 2023). Anti-ableist feminist social movement organizations, like Las FemiDiskas, are among the actors in this broader feminist environment that are developing virtual engagement strategies to fight against the ableist and sexist violence endured in both private and public spaces (Murillo Lafuente, 2023). These endeavors make it clear that women with disabilities are not taking lying down but instead are actively fighting against patriarchal violence, especially in the Global South.

Although there is no extensive documentation about youth-led initiatives for disability resistance in Latin America within the literature provided, such initiatives are usually defined by the creative and innovative usage of social media and new technologies for civic engagement and collective action (Lupien, 2020). In this light, young disabled activists will probably utilize the same means as their peers, thus taking a digital route for raising awareness, protest organizing, and building solidarity, especially in the context of limited access to political participation through traditional means. The case of the COVID-19 pandemic is, for instance, one that brought to the surface the plight of people with disabilities in Mexico, as lockdowns revealed problems of boredom and isolation, which, in turn, might have led to artistic and activist responses among the youth (Miranda-Galarza & Mayer-Foulkes, 2023).

5.4.4 Transnational and Cross-Border Solidarities

Transnational solidarity has been a recurrent practice in Latin America from the very beginning, primarily through leftist groups and human rights campaigns (Churchill, 2009; Hatzky & Stites Mor, 2014; Riethof & Smith, 2023). This kind of solidarity means that the distant or unequal groups cooperate with each other, thus gaining political resources that are very important for their social and political change (Hatzky & Stites Mor, 2014). For disability resistance movements, alliances across borders and even globally become indispensable for their messages to be heard and rights to be advocated for internationally (Meekosha, 2011). The Inter-American Solidarity and Cooperation Declaration of 1936, for example, was aimed at integrating the region and therefore set a precedent for cooperative endeavors in the Americas (Bailliet, 2023).

In recent times, connectivity across nations has proven to be still important. Take, for example, the feminist groups in Latin America that are protesting with global movements like "Global Iran," thus showing how solidarity transcends not only borders but also identity lines (Louie, 2025). There is a reconfiguration of North–South solidarity being called for, a reflection on how power relations in a country like the U.S. affect its solidarity ties with Latin America (Sundberg, 2007). This is interpreted as equitable partnerships being required for rehabilitation and disability rights advocacy, where the distinct needs and capacities of the Global South communities are recognized (Marshall et al., 2004; Padilla, 2023). Indigenous activists from different countries have been fighting for self-direction, at times making national governments grant them concessions, which, though still facing implementation challenges, can be strengthened by international backing and transnational advocacy networks (Rayo et al., 2024). The impact of the Convention on the Rights of Persons with Disabilities, although constrained by its limitations, has nonetheless been responsible for sounding the rights-based claim and political incidence bell anew all over the Latin America region by disability movements (Rebolledo-Sanhueza & Galaz-Valderrama, 2024).

The disability resistance movements in Latin America consist of a wide variety of groups that mirror and directly reflect the social, cultural, and political complexities of the entire region. Besides, the movements are marked by such elements as the intense focus on the self-determination of indigenous and Afro-descendant peoples, the significant presence of women- and youth-led initiatives, and the increasing importance of transnational solidarities in confronting ableism and advocating for the rights of people with disabilities and for inclusive societies (Lapierre, 2023; Murillo Lafuente, 2023; Padilla, 2023; Pino-Morán et al., 2023; Rebolledo-Sanhueza & Galaz-Valderrama, 2024).

5.5 Protest, Direct Action, and Public Space

In Latin America, the monumental landscape of disability activism is marked by protests, direct actions, and the reclaiming of public spaces, which have led to controversies between state institutions and the colonial past. The constant through line to this activism was the intertwining of indigenous traditions and the collective embodiment of disability; thus, making the forms of resistance unique (Brégain et al., 2022; Lapierre, 2023).

In the case of Latin America, disability activism has found its ways into streets, land occupations, and even sacred spaces Disability movements in Latin America often resort to the use of public spaces for protest as a means of expressing their demands, which is in line with the history of social movements in the region that used streets and plazas to voice grievances and demand rights. For example, in Bolivia, disability activists carried out big protests, most of which included the occupation of public spaces, so they could get allowances and their rights recognized more. A similar case has been observed in the case of Chile, where large protesters have branded Telethon as a charity model rather than a rights-based approach in the field and thus are attempting to challenge it (Brégain et al., 2022). These actions result in the transformation of the usually passive public spaces into arenas where political assertion occurs by the mere physical presence of people with disabilities, which challenges the societal norms and the visibility.

The public space concept beyond city areas includes tribal lands and sacred places, especially for natives. While the literature does not elaborate much on land occupations or protests in sacred places with a focus on disabled persons, the wider context of indigenous resistance in Latin America gives a basis for such possible mobilizations to be understood. The indigenous people often interpret disability according to their religious beliefs and cultural habits, which may include traditional healing and community support systems that are opposed to the Western medical model (Lapierre, 2023). The fight for ancestral lands and cultural preservation among indigenous groups, like those living on Nicaragua's Caribbean Coast, who organize against land encroachment, is nothing but reclaiming and defending their "public" and sacred territories (Guillen, 2022). These movements, though not solely disability-focused, have created places where disability is present and can be dealt with through a culturally appropriate resistance framework.

Indigenous protest traditions and collective embodiment of disability in Latin America. Indigenous protest traditions in Latin America are very much tied to the historical struggles against colonialism, forced assimilation, and political violence.

These traditions are often characterized by collective actions that highlight community solidarity and the connection to the ancestors' heritage. The indigenous people with disabilities find in these very traditions a powerful means of describing their experiences and making their demands. Disability, through the movements, is considered the "collective embodiment," which, in this case, is a total rejection of the individualistic Western conceptualization of disability, and instead, the communal identity and shared struggle are adopted. In this setting, disability is regarded as an additional aspect of the historical marginalization that has been suffered by the indigenous communities, entwined with race, poverty, and land rights (Lapierre, 2023).

The blending of disability activism into the larger picture of indigenous movements is using the already established structures of resistance and the traditional modes of protest to the fullest. Political mobilization among Afro-descendant peoples in Latin America, based on issues like racial discrimination and cultural identity, has been continually boosted by the acknowledgment of multicultural characteristics in modern societies (Agudelo, 2010). Just as indigenous disability collectives, while working in their own unique cultural settings, are able to employ well-established indigenous protest tactics to gain attention for their specific needs, such as access to culturally sensitive healthcare and resources, so are the indigenous disability groups (Lapierre, 2023).

Challenging state institutions and the development of disability in Latin America. A crucial aspect of disability resistance movements in Latin America is to directly confront government institutions and the often-exclusionary character of development projects (Brégain et al., 2022). The Convention on the Rights of Persons with Disabilities (CRPD) has been a key tool in prompting these movements to assert their rights and claim political power, despite its limitations in practice (Rebolledo-Sanhueza & Galaz-Valderrama, 2024). Activists frequently point their fingers at government policies that bring about less social aid, non-accessibility, and discrimination as the root cause of the problems.

In the case of Argentina, activists have taken their protests against the implementation of drastic cuts to disability benefits and services, which can be viewed as a direct confrontation of state policies that have an impact on the lives of disabled people (Brégain et al., 2022). These protests bring to the fore the conflict between state-led initiatives, which at times adopt a medical or charitable model of disability, and the rights-based advocacy of disability activists who demand full integration and equal opportunities.

In addition, development projects, even if at the surface they are trying to bring about progress, may somehow or directly harm the communities, the disabled ones among others, via disrupting their customary ways of living, evicting people, or just not meeting the accessibility standards set. The struggles of maroon communities, descendants of fugitives from slavery, in pursuing political goals through the production and mobilization of space, illustrate a long history of resistance against dominant societal structures that have historically excluded them (Guillen, 2022). The very existence of these groups and their claims to the territory implicitly or explicitly confront the prevailing development models not only in terms of their interests but also including the disabled members of the communities.

The pandemic of COVID-19 was a revelation of the enormous problems that disabled people in Mexico had to deal with, especially with regard to isolation and confinement, that was the case, and the result of it was a series of artistic and activist responses which indirectly had the effect of making the government re-evaluate its responses to the crisis through the engagement of public discourse (Miranda-Galarza & Mayer-Foulkes, 2023). It was a period that exposed the continuous marginalization of disabled people and the necessity for advocacy to be very strong to ensure that disabled people are not neglected in times of crisis or development projects. Disability resistance movements in Latin America are dynamic and multi-faceted, employing methods such as direct action, occupying public and symbolic spaces, and embedding their struggles within broader indigenous and sociopolitical contexts to overcome systemic ableism and advocate for a more inclusive society.

5.6 Digital Activism-Based Modern Platforms on Disability in Latin America

In Latin America, digital activism and modern tools have come to be the very necessary means of disability movements, obtaining much better visibility through social media and building alliances at the same time they were dealing with the issues of accessibility, language fairness, and digital divides that still exist (Lupien, 2020). These platforms are not only places for sharing stories but also for supporting global advocacy, thus having the potential to significantly impact the conversation and mobilization around the rights of disabled people.

Social media as a Tool for Visibility and Coalition-Building on Disability in Latin America: The use of social media platforms has gained the status of essential instruments for disability movements in Latin America, where they have also brought in visibility and the strengthening of alliances. Among the groups that are on the margins of society as persons with disabilities, who in most cases are excluded from the media and public discourse, social networks give an easy and fast way to express their life stories and state their claims (Lupien, 2020). All this is particularly important in an area where conventional media might not cover disability topics well or might even perpetuate the stereotypical portrayals.

Activists make use of Twitter, Facebook, Instagram, and other platforms to inform the public, to arrange campaigns, and to highlight the issues of systemic ableism and violations of human rights (Murillo Lafuente, 2023). By the way, Las FemiDiskas—a feminist, anti-ableist, social movement organization—has managed to make good use of virtual engagement strategies to bring about an end to and/or resist the violence inflicted on women and especially black women in the Global South due to ableism and sexism. This shows the powerful ability of digital tools for activists, creating a safe space for discussion and collective action, overcoming the physical barriers and geographical distances that would otherwise limit mobilization.

Moreover, social media plays a role in the very quick building of coalitions, which helps various groups to get together around the same goal (Lupien, 2020). One of the outcomes is a kind of alliance between disability and other social justice activists, which, among others, are indigenous rights, Afro-descendant communities, and feminist organizations. The cross-sharing of narratives and resources between the different movements not only lets them become more powerful as their membership increases, but it also creates a more unified front against systemic inequalities. In the same way, the use of hashtags and the going viral nature of campaigns can make local issues get to the national and even international level very quickly, thus putting a lot of pressure on the government and institutions to pay more attention to and be more effective in addressing disability rights.

Accessibility, Language Justice, and Digital Divides on Disability in Latin America: The advent of digital platforms to a certain extent changed the methodology for disability activism in Latin America; however, the accessibility aspect together with language justice and digital divides still being the main problems, the activists have to face the significant hurdles mentioned. The major problem is the lack of accessibility, which is an inherent characteristic of many digital platforms and of online content altogether, thus preventing, among others, invention with and participation of persons with sensory, motor, or cognitive disabilities. For instance, the usage of shapes in website designs, the prohibition of video captions, or the addition of complex features can discourage the participation of disabled people in online activism to the extent that they will be removed entirely from this process. The problem of accessibility goes as far as crisis information, where people with disabilities are cut off from the complex digital platforms during disasters, leading to a situation that is already life-threatening, becoming even more so (Kent & Ellis, 2015).

Language justice is another cornerstone of the issue at hand, especially in a region that has the richest in the world variety of languages, and even among the indigenous languages. The use of the main languages such as Spanish and Portuguese in the content that is primarily targeted to the dominant language speakers can be seen as turning an ever-wider gap between the states and the indigenous communities plus other groups who prefer their non-native languages for the communication, thereby aggravating and at the same time limiting their participation in the digital policy as a result of the advocating of the languages and the making-matter-oneself-heard. The very cultural characteristics and outlooks associated with disability in the indigenous context often stand in contrast to the Western viewpoint; it is absolutely necessary to have the online presence of the linguistic and cultural diversity acknowledged and respected (Lapierre, 2023).

The digital divide makes the whole situation even more difficult. Reliable internet, devices that are not so expensive, and the know-how of using digital tools are still not evenly spread out throughout Latin America, with the latter ones being the ones mostly affected. While social media opens up new ways for people to get involved in civic activities, the fact that it is so dependent on the internet means that many people at the bottom of the hierarchy do not have the chance to join the online movements or get hold of important information (Lupien, 2020). This situation indicates that the traditional methods, such as protests and direct actions, will continue to be important for many communities despite the availability of digital tools.

Online Storytelling and Transnational Advocacy on Disability in Latin America: In the digital era, online storytelling is nothing short of a revolution and has become a major force in the lives of disability rights advocates in Latin America, as they have no option but to fight for their existence, topple misconceptions, and gain audiences for their causes. Through blogging, personal testimonies, video, and social media posts, people with disabilities disclose their daily lives as well as feelings and thoughts, thus arousing empathy and comprehension of the wider audience (Murillo Lafuente, 2023). This direct narrative style opposes the usually dehumanizing medical or charitable models of disability that the court isn't even truthful to, advocating instead a rights-based viewpoint where inclusivity and equality are the very essence of the universe (Rebolledo-Sanhueza & Galaz-Valderrama, 2024).

These individual accounts, more often than not, go beyond the geographical boundaries of a nation, thus aiding in the transnational advocacy campaigns. The storytelling over the internet by the disabled activists in Latin America leads to connecting with the worldwide movements for disabled people, paving the way for finding allies and getting support from international friends (Padilla, 2023). The transnational aspect is crucial to the cause as it not only helps to make their voices heard but also to influence the global policy talks on the rights of disabled people 5. To illustrate, the UN Convention on the Rights of Persons with Disabilities (CRPD) has given a new lease of life to the rights claims and political incidence of the disability movements in Latin America, where the online platforms are doing most of the work in sharing the good and bad experiences related to its implementation (Rebolledo-Sanhueza & Galaz-Valderrama, 2024).

The term "fugitive, maroon knowledges and global south epistemologies" seems to fit the situation very well since the Internet spaces enable the promotion of non-Western and even opposite-to-the-Western understandings and solutions for the disability issue that are not only Western narratives. These online places are gifts for the movements doing cross-coalitional building, as they not only unite anti-racist and anti-ableist movements in the Global North but also in the Global South (Padilla, 2023). The experiences of disabled persons during the COVID-19 pandemic have been an eye-opener, showing how the affiliated issues like confinement and boredom, especially in Mexico, can be turned by the online platforms into artistic and activist responses that not only engage with the public discourse but also foster connections even when physical isolation is present (Miranda-Galarza & Mayer-Foulkes, 2023).

Ultimately, digital activism in Latin America is a very active and still developing area of practice, which not only provides a great deal of power to the rights of disabled people's movements but also asks for workflows and strategies to keep on dealing with accessibility, language, and digital inclusion problems to make sure that everyone can participate.

5.7 Challenges and Tensions Within Decolonial Disability Activisms

Decolonized disability activism in Latin America has to deal with a number of complicated issues and tensions that are all connected to the historical problem of colonialism, together with its aftermath of ableism and socio-economic inequality. These activities try to get rid of the disabled people's perspective conceived in the West and want to be recognized as rights not just in the West but also according to their own culture that might be different from the West and thus they are in conflict with the integration of the various ways of perceiving things, the limits of international legal instruments, and the constantly growing digital and socio-economic gap (Lapierre, 2023; Padilla, 2023; Rebolledo-Sanhueza & Galaz-Valderrama, 2024).

The biggest problem is trying to bring together different worldviews and experiences of disability. For example, the indigenous groups of Latin America deal with disability according to their own culture and religion, which is usually quite a distance from the Western medical or individualistic models of disability. This view of the indigenous people is often patient-centered and emphasizes healing through their natives and not through a doctor's clinic. So, the conflict arises when the decolonial disability activism, which is ant-Western and relies on global perspectives to define disability rights and shape the Convention on the Rights of Persons with Disabilities (CRPD), tries to incorporate these different indigenous views at the same time as engaging with a broader disability rights discourse that is dominating by the global North and the CRPD (Padilla, 2023; Rebolledo-Sanhueza & Galaz-Valderrama, 2024; Velarde, 2018). It is "language justice," and the task is "difficult" to make sure that the different voices not only get to be heard but get to be integrated into the advocacy efforts authentically, as the dominant languages like Spanish and Portuguese can unintentionally sidestep the indigenous people's linguistic and conceptual frameworks, thus causing (Velarde, 2018).

One more area of friction is the issue of international legal frameworks such as the CRPD. Even though the CRPD had been a significant factor in the rights claiming movements and political empowerment across Latin America, its execution still encounters considerable restrictions, especially at the national and local levels. The limitations arise due to many reasons, such as a lack of political interest, a lack of funding, and the complex nature of applying the concept of universal rights in the case of different cultures and socio-economic backgrounds. Decolonial perspectives question how such global regulations, even though ambitious, sometimes unintentionally impose the same universalizing view, especially on the Global South's specific historical and cultural realities. Activists are often put at risk; they are using the CRPD for advocacy while at the same time demanding local, decolonized interpretations and implementations of disability and justice (Rebolledo-Sanhueza & Galaz-Valderrama, 2024).

Besides that, the ongoing socio-economic and digital gaps are tremendous obstacles for the decolonization of disability activist movements. In Latin America, there are still extreme inequalities in terms of access to resources, education, and technology that mainly affect the marginalized groups, including persons with disabilities, indigenous populations, and Afro-descendants (Hooker, 2008; Lapierre, 2023; Paschel & Sawyer, 2008). The "digital divide" indicates that while social media provides new avenues for visibility and alliance-building, many disabled people living in rural or economically disadvantaged areas do not have access to the internet, affordable devices, and are not trained in digital skills, thus preventing them from participating in online activism (Lupien, 2020). On one hand, there is the creation of a situation where digital platforms, which were supposed to encourage equal participation in advocacy, may, in fact, because of the existing inequalities, cut off the most marginalized groups. On the other hand, the socio-economic conditions, i.e., high poverty indexes associated with the indigenous people, lead to more difficulties faced by disabled people, making the accessibility of basic services and support a more urgent issue than the legal rights, which are mainly existential (Lapierre, 2023).

The idea of cross-coalitional building is also fraught with contradictions. It is clear that there is a need to ally the anti-racist with the anti-ableist movement, plus to tap into "fugitive, maroon knowledges and global south epistemologies" (Padilla, 2023), but the joining of these various struggles is hard to do. Discrimination in its various forms and degrees, be it based on race, ethnicity, or class, very often overlaps with disability, thus giving rise to multiple layers of marginalization (Hooker, 2008; Lapierre, 2023). Decolonial disability activism must take great care not to lose the particular experiences of Afro-descendants with disabilities, for instance, in the thick of the more general categories, but, rather, to have them recognized in their distinctive complexity (Hooker, 2008). All this will need the constant involvement and acknowledgment of the different groups in the society that are being oppressed, so that the hierarchies within the liberation movements are not unintentionally sustained, and hence the dialogue does not become a monopoly of the stronger parts in the society.

To sum up, the battles of declaring and preserving the independence of such movements against state structures or mainstream development are very much alive. Protests in Argentina against the reduced mobility of the state in the disability sector are a reminder of the ongoing struggle with the state, which often has to choose between cutting down on social welfare. Decolonial disability activism takes a step further in contesting the very social and political structures that unite them, yet at the same time, they have to make these structures their partners while securing grants and making policy changes. This type of partnership comes with a possibility of the radicals' demands being diluted or the whole movement being swallowed by the existing ones, which are often ableist. In this regard, a critique of the Telethon in Chile, which some regard as perpetuating a charity model rather than a rights-based approach, is a good example of this tension (Brégain et al., 2022).

To put it differently, decoupling or decolonizing disability activism in Latin America cannot be seen merely as a struggle but rather as a sustained effort through the various themes of the struggle to redefine, with the point of view that acknowledges and respects the local hierarchies of knowledge, to unsettle the colonial structures, and to build inclusive movements, all the while dealing with the root of the problem of profound social inequalities and the intricacies of the global and local power relations.

5.8 Conclusion

The Latin American indigenous and decolonial disability activism is a radical break with the colonial logic, which has always attached negative connotations like deficit, pathology, or social burden to disability. The activists of these movements do not want to get simple inclusion in the already existing systems; instead, they want a total transformation of society, its values, institutions, and epistemologies. Decolonial disability activism brings attention to the Indigenous knowledge, relationships, land, and community care, which start to show the power of coloniality and ability that still determine the valuation of bodies and the death of lives. In this scenario, disability is not a single condition but rather a living experience that is very much tied up with the interconnectedness of colonial violence, racial capitalism, environmental dispossession, gender oppression, and state neglect. The chapter highlights that resistance has many faces: community organizing, protest, art, storytelling, digital advocacy, and transnational solidarity, each of which is deeply rooted in the local histories and struggles but at the same time is able to resonate across borders. These activisms, however, maintain the demand for epistemic justice: knowledge concerning disabilities must originate from the disabled indigenous folk, in their own languages, cultural frameworks, and political terms. The chapter does not shy away from mentioning the existing tensions, such as the engagement with the CRPD, not so much the 'global rights frameworks', which, among other sources of conflict, may give rise to hierarchies inside the movements and the structural inequalities that restrict access to resources and digital spaces. To sum it up, the Indigenous and decolonial disability movements put forth the idea of making a transition from claiming rights to assuming responsibility, from looking at the disabled persons only as producers to being the receivers of the privileges, and finally from seeing individuals as independent to recognizing their interdependence for survival. Latin America can never be considered a separate continent when it comes to the fight for disability justice because it is the same case as with land, sovereignty, racial justice, and decolonization struggles. By that, these movements not only provide ways of resistance but also the future by which people will be treated according to their rights, and that is by being interdependent and self-determined.

References

Agudelo, C. (2010). Movilizaciones afrodescendientes en América Latina Una visión panorámica de algunas experiencias contra la exclusión y por el derecho a la identidad. *Colombia Internacional*, (71), 109–126. https://doi.org/10.7440/colombiaint71.2010.06

Arroyo-Rojas, F. (2024). Unpacking ableism: Perspectives from the Chilean physical education discourse. *Kinesiology Review, 13*(3), 376–382. https://doi.org/10.1123/kr.2024-0014

Bailliet, C. M. (2023, January). The role of solidarity as an international right and duty within Latin America. In *Proceedings of the ASIL Annual Meeting* (Vol. 117, pp. 107–109). Cambridge University Press.

Berthelot-Raffard, A. (2024). From capacitalism to disability justice in academia: A philosophical manifesto. *Equity in Education & Society*. https://doi.org/10.1177/27526461241307326

Boda, P. A., Nusbaum, E. A., & Kulkarni, S. S. (2022). From 'what is' toward 'what if' through intersectionality: Problematizing ableist erasures and coloniality in racially just research. *International Journal of Research & Method in Education, 45*(4), 356–369. https://doi.org/10.25417/uic.21526167

Brégain, G., Venturiello, M. P., Ferrante, C., & Fuente-Alba, L. V. (2022). Les actions protestataires des personnes handicapées en Bolivie, au Chili et en Argentine. *Canadian Journal of Latin American and Caribbean Studies/revue Canadienne des Études Latino-Américaines Et Caraïbes, 47*(3), 369–389. https://doi.org/10.1080/08263663.2022.2110746

Campos, C. R. R. (2021). Inequality, social mobility, and racism in Bolivia. In *The Oxford handbook of the sociology of Latin America* (p. 177).

Capella Palacios, M., & Jadhav, S. (2020). How coloniality shapes the making of Latin American psychologists: Ethnographic evidence from Ecuador. *International Review of Psychiatry, 32*(4), 348–358. https://doi.org/10.1080/09540261.2020.1761777

Churchill, L. (2009). Transnational alliances: Radical US feminist solidarity and contention with Latin America, 1970–1989. *Latin American Perspectives, 36*(6), 10–26. https://doi.org/10.1177/0094582X09350761

da Nóbrega Rogoski, B., Caldas, R. C. S., Souza Guevara, V. L. D., Louzeiro, R., Vasconcelos, L. A., & Flores, E. P. (2024). Autism activism movement in Brazil: Contingency analysis and the Pacto pela Neurodiversidade (Pledge for Neurodiversity). *Trends in Psychology*, 1–20. https://doi.org/10.1007/s43076-024-00406-y

Daniels-Mayes, S. (2023). Researching Indigenous people living with a disability: The urgent need for an intersectional and decolonising approach (BlakAbility). *First Nations Health and Wellbeing-the Lowitja Journal, 1*, Article 100004. https://doi.org/10.1016/j.fnhli.2023.100004

de Lima Costa, C. (2020). Latin America, decoloniality, and translation: Feminists building connectant epistemologies. https://doi.org/10.1093/oso/9780190062965.003.0011

Ferrari, M. B. (2020). Feminismos descoloniales y discapacidad: hacia una conceptualización de la colonialidad de la capacidad. *Nómadas*, (52), 115–131. https://doi.org/10.30578/nomadas.n52a7

Gandarilla Salgado, J. G., García-Bravo, M. H., & Benzi, D. (2021). Two decades of Anibal Quijano's coloniality of power, Eurocentrism and Latin America. *Contexto Internacional, 43*, 199–222. https://doi.org/10.1590/s0102-8529.2019430100009

Gibson, S. (2012). Narrative accounts of university education: Socio-cultural perspectives of students with disabilities. *Disability & Society, 27*(3), 353–369. https://doi.org/10.1080/09687599.2012.654987

Gilroy, J., Dew, A., Lincoln, M., Ryall, L., Jensen, H., Taylor, K., Barton, R., McRae, K., & Flood, V. (2018). Indigenous persons with disability in remote Australia: Research methodology and Indigenous community control. *Disability & Society, 33*(7), 1025–1045. https://doi.org/10.1080/09687599.2018.1478802

Grech, S. (2017). Decolonising Eurocentric disability studies: Why colonialism matters in the disability and global South debate. In *Disability and colonialism* (pp. 6–21). Routledge. https://doi.org/10.1080/13504630.2014.995347

Guillen, A. L. Z. (2022). Maroon socioterritorial movements. *Annals of the American Association of Geographers, 112*(4), 1123–1138. https://doi.org/10.1080/24694452.2021.1959293

Hatzky, C., & Stites Mor, J. (2014). Latin American transnational solidarities: Contexts and critical research paradigms. *Journal of Iberian and Latin American Research, 20*(2), 127–140. https://doi.org/10.1080/13260219.2014.939121

Hollinsworth, D. (2013). Decolonizing indigenous disability in Australia. *Disability & Society, 28*(5), 601–615. https://doi.org/10.1080/09687599.2012.717879

Hooker, J. (2008). Afro-descendant struggles for collective rights in Latin America: Between race and culture. *Souls, 10*(3), 279–291. https://doi.org/10.1080/10999940802347764

Horta, Í. B., Saraiva, A. M. A., & Torres, J. P. (2023). A emergência da interseccionalidade nos debates sobre deficiência: contribuições de pensamentos decoloniais latino-americanos. *Revista Relicário.*

Hutcheon, E. J., & Lashewicz, B. (2020). Tracing and troubling continuities between ableism and colonialism in Canada. *Disability & Society, 35*(5), 695–714. https://doi.org/10.1080/09687599.2019.1647145

Hutcheon, E., & Lashewicz, B. (2014). Theorizing resilience: Critiquing and unbounding a marginalizing concept. *Disability & Society, 29*(9), 1383–1397. https://doi.org/10.1080/09687599.2014.934954

Jantzen, W. (2015). Inklusion und Kolonialität-Gegenrede zu einer unpolitischen Inklusionsdebatte. *Jahrbuch Für Pädagogik, 2015*(1), 241–253. https://doi.org/10.3726/267059_241

Kallio-Tavin, M., & Wexler, A. (2022). Decentering colonialism and ableism in artistic practices. *Research in Arts and Education, 2022*(3), 5–16. https://doi.org/10.54916/rae.125081

Kent, M., & Ellis, K. (2015). People with disability and new disaster communications: Access and the social media mash-up. *Disability & Society, 30*(3), 419–431. https://doi.org/10.1080/09687599.2015.1021756

King, J. A., Brough, M., & Knox, M. (2014). Negotiating disability and colonisation: The lived experience of indigenous Australians with a disability. *Disability & Society, 29*(5), 738–750. https://doi.org/10.1080/09687599.2013.864257

Lapierre, M. (2023). Disability and Latin American indigenous peoples. *Disability & Society, 38*(7), 1276–1280. https://doi.org/10.1080/09687599.2023.2192381

Leal, N. M. O., & Torres, C. P. M. (2024). Una Mirada a la Normatividad Latinoamericana en la Inclusión de Personas con Discapacidad. *Ciencia Latina Revista Científica Multidisciplinar*, *8*(2), 4918–4938. https://doi.org/10.37811/cl_rcm.v8i2.10907

León, J. J. P. (2024). Popular and decolonial veganism: Animal Rights, racialized and indigenous subjectivities in Latin America. *Relations: Beyond Anthropocentrism, 12*, 49. https://doi.org/10.7358/rela-2024-01-ponj

Louie, E. (2025). Crossing borders and connecting feminists: "Global Iran" and solidarity protests in Latin America. *Digest of Middle East Studies, 34*(4), Article e70006. https://doi.org/10.1111/dome.70006

Lupien, P. (2020). Indigenous movements, collective action, and social media: New opportunities or new threats?. *Social Media+ Society*, *6*(2). https://doi.org/10.1177/2056305120926487

Lyra, L. (2023). On women, pans, and politics: Imagining decolonial gendered urban spatialities. *Urban Geography, 44*(9), 1951–1972. https://doi.org/10.1080/02723638.2023.2238566

MacKeigan, T. (2021). Sexual citizenship through resistance: A movement that centers disabled women's voices. *Disability & Society, 36*(4), 656–677. https://doi.org/10.1080/09687599.2020.1751077

Marshall, C. A., Burross, H. L., Gotto, G., McAllan, L., Martínez, P. V., Juárez, L. G., & Rey, P. F. (2004). The United States and Mexico: Creating partnerships in rehabilitation. *Rehabilitation Psychology, 49*(1), 14. https://doi.org/10.1037/0090-5550.49.1.14

Medina, M. C. (2023). The feminization of resistance: The narratives of# NiUnaMenos as social transformative action. *Journal of Political Power, 16*(2), 237–253. https://doi.org/10.1080/2158379X.2023.2251109

Meekosha, H. (2011). Decolonising disability: Thinking and acting globally. *Disability & Society, 26*(6), 667–682. https://doi.org/10.1080/09687599.2011.602860

Mendoza, B. (2015). Coloniality of gender and power. In *The Oxford handbook of feminist theory* (pp. 100–121). https://doi.org/10.1093/oxfordhb/9780199328581.013.6

Miranda-Galarza, B., & Mayer-Foulkes, B. (2023). Boredom, art, and activism: Notes on the experiences of people with disabilities in Mexico during the COVID-19 pandemic. *Frontiers in Sociology, 8*, 1215106. https://doi.org/10.3389/fsoc.2023.1215106

Montiel Valle, D. (2021). Unearthing neoliberal multiculturalism in news discourse: Politics of indigeneity & ethnic identity in Nicaragua's Caribbean Coast. *Critical Studies in Media Communication, 38*(4), 350–364. https://doi.org/10.1080/15295036.2021.1945119

Moura Jr, J. F., de Sousa Lima, A. A., Portela, F. F., Lisboa, S. J., Carvalho, T. S., Pitaguary, R., & Kaninde, J. A. J. (2024). The indigenous foundations of decolonial community psychology. In *Handbook of decolonial community psychology* (pp. 531–542). Springer Nature Switzerland. https://doi.org/10.1007/978-3-031-67035-0_29

Murillo Lafuente, I. E. (2023). Spaces of anti-ableist, feminist resistance. *Space and Culture, 26*(3), 433–450. https://doi.org/10.1177/12063312231181529

Ortega, D. C. V. (2023). Tierra de imbunches y ch'uqtas: la dis-capacidad como dispositivo colonial en América Latina y el Caribe. *Brazilian Journal of Latin American Studies, 22*(47), 197–222. https://doi.org/10.11606/issn.1676-6288.prolam.23.213227

Padilla, A. (2023). Cross-coalitional anti-racist and anti-ableist movements? Building on maroon/fugitive knowledges and global south epistemologies. *Disability Studies Quarterly, 43*(1). https://doi.org/10.18061/dsq.v43i1.9660

Paschel, T. S., & Sawyer, M. Q. (2008). Contesting politics as usual: Black social movements, globalization, and race policy in Latin America. *Souls, 10*(3), 197–214. https://doi.org/10.1080/10999940802347707

Pestka, K., & Wendt, S. (2014). Belonging: Women living with intellectual disabilities and experiences of domestic violence. *Disability & Society, 29*(7), 1031–1045. https://doi.org/10.1080/09687599.2014.902358

Pinilla-Roncancio, M., & Rodríguez Caicedo, N. (2022). Legislation on disability and employment: To what extent are employment rights guaranteed for persons with disabilities? *International Journal of Environmental Research and Public Health, 19*(9), 5654. https://doi.org/10.3390/ijerph19095654

Pino-Morán, J. A., Rodríguez-Garrido, P., Zango-Martín, I., & Mora-Malo, E. (2022). Discursos políticos de activistas disidentes de la discapacidad en Chile. *Revista De Estudios Sociales,* (81), 3–20. https://doi.org/10.7440/res81.2022.01

Pino-Morán, J. A., Zango-Martin, I., Rodríguez-Garrido, P., & Mora-Malo, E. (2023). Reivindicative occupational practices of activist with disabilities. *Cadernos Brasileiros De Terapia Ocupacional, 31*, Article e3510. https://doi.org/10.1590/2526-8910.ctoao269135102

Puszka, S., Walsh, C., Markham, F., Barney, J., Yap, M., & Dreise, T. (2022). Towards the decolonisation of disability: A systematic review of disability conceptualisations, practices and experiences of First Nations people of Australia. *Social Science & Medicine, 305*, Article 115047. https://doi.org/10.1016/j.socscimed.2022.115047

Quijano, A. (2016). 'Bien Vivir'–between 'Development' and the De/coloniality of Power. *Alternautas (Re) Searching Development: The Abya Yala Chapter*, *3*(1), 10–23. https://doi.org/10.31273/alternautas.v3i1.1023

Rayo, G. A., Mosinger, E. S., & Thaler, K. M. (2024). Statebuilding and indigenous rights implementation: Political incentives, social movement pressure, and autonomy policy in Central America. *World Development, 175*, Article 106468. https://doi.org/10.1016/j.worlddev.2023.106468

Rebolledo-Sanhueza, J. A., & Galaz-Valderrama, C. (2024). Activismo y discapacidad en Latinoamérica: luchas por el reconocimiento. *Revista Estudos Feministas*, *32*(1). https://doi.org/10.1590/1806-9584-2024v32n190769

Rice, C., Dion, S. D., & Chandler, E. (2021). Decolonizing disability through activist art, *41*(2). https://doi.org/10.18061/dsq.v41i2.7130

Riethof, M., & Smith, R. G. (2023). Researching Latin America in liverpool: Transnational connections of hope and solidarity. *Bulletin of Hispanic Studies, 100*(10), 1079–1093. https://doi.org/10.3828/bhs.2023.73

Rivas Velarde, M., (2018) Indigenous perspectives of disability. *Disability Studies Quarterly, 38*(4). https://doi.org/10.18061/dsq.v38i4.6114

Rodríguez, I., & Inturias, M. L. (2018). Conflict transformation in indigenous peoples' territories: Doing environmental justice with a 'decolonial turn.' *Development Studies Research, 5*(1), 90–105. https://doi.org/10.1080/21665095.2018.1486220

Rodríguez-Garrido, P., & Pino-Morán, J. A. (2023). Motherhood, disability, and rurality: Descolonising practices and knowledge via the Las Quiscas case in Chile. *Gender & Development, 31*(2–3), 361–381. https://doi.org/10.1080/13552074.2023.2254570

Roy, A. (2024). Decolonizing disability studies: Identities, epistemologies and global south perspectives. *The Creative Launcher*, *9*(6), 70–81. https://doi.org/10.53032/tcl.2024.9.6.07

Salvatore, R. D. (2010). The postcolonial in Latin America and the concept of coloniality: A historian's point of view. *A Contracorriente: Una revista de estudios latinoamericanos, 8*(1), 332–348. www.ncsu.edu/project/acontracorriente

Schilling-Vacaflor, A., & Flemmer, R. (2020). Mobilising free, prior and informed consent (FPIC) from below: A typology of indigenous peoples' agency. *International Journal on Minority and Group Rights, 27*(2), 291–313. https://doi.org/10.1163/15718115-02702008

Sepúlveda Jara, R., & Oyarce Pisani, A. M. (2020). New and old knowledge aimed at decolonising mental health: Reflections and proposals from Chile. *International Review of Psychiatry*, *32*(4), 334–339. https://doi.org/10.1080/09540261.2020.1767042

Setio, R. (2025). Decolonizing disability in social and theology structures: An Indonesian perspective1. *Journal of Disability & Religion*, 1–19. https://doi.org/10.1080/23312521.2025.2531798

Shekha, K. R. (2011). Determinants of Latin American activism: Domestic and transnational political opportunities and threats. *Sociology Compass, 5*(8), 747–762. https://doi.org/10.1111/j.1751-9020.2011.00396.x

Strawn, K. D. (2009). Contemporary research on social movements and protest in Latin America: Promoting democracy, resisting neoliberalism, and many themes in between. *Sociology Compass, 3*(4), 644–657. https://doi.org/10.1111/j.1751-9020.2009.00217.x

Sundberg, J. (2007). Reconfiguring north–south solidarity: Critical reflections on experiences of transnational resistance. *Antipode, 39*(1), 144–166. https://doi.org/10.1111/j.1467-8330.2007.00510.x

Valenzuela, C. G. (2023). Disrupting curricula and pedagogies in Latin American universities: six criteria for decolonising the university. In *Possibilities and Complexities of Decolonising Higher Education* (pp. 133–151). Routledge. https://doi.org/10.4324/9781003373827

Van Cott, D. L. (2005). Building inclusive democracies: Indigenous peoples and ethnic minorities in Latin America. *Democratisation, 12*(5), 820–837. https://doi.org/10.1080/13510340500322215

Vaughan, C., Khaw, S., Katsikis, G., Wheeler, J., Ozge, J., Kasidis, V., & Moosad, L. (2019). 'It is like being put through a blender': Inclusive research in practice in an Australian university. *Disability & Society, 34*(7–8), 1224–1240. https://doi.org/10.1080/09687599.2019.1603103

Velarde, M. R. (2018). Indigenous perspectives of disability. *Disability Studies Quarterly*, *38*(4). https://doi.org/10.18061/dsq.v38i4.6114

Waterfield, B., Beagan, B. B., & Weinberg, M. (2018). Disabled academics: A case study in Canadian universities. *Disability & Society, 33*(3), 327–348. https://doi.org/10.1080/09687599.2017.1411251

Woods, R., Milton, D., Arnold, L., & Graby, S. (2018). Redefining critical autism studies: A more inclusive interpretation. *Disability & Society, 33*(6), 974–979. https://doi.org/10.1080/09687599.2018.1454380

Yellowhorse, S. (2022). Disability and indigenous resistance: Mapping value politics during the time of COVID-19. *AlterNative: An International Journal of Indigenous Peoples*, *18*(4), 605–612. https://doi.org/10.1177/11771801221123328

Chapter 6
Toward a Decolonial Politics of Disability Justice in Latin America

Abstract A critical evaluation of the current understanding of disability leads this segment to propose a decolonial politics of disability justice in Latin America, which has been precipitated by the scrutiny of the colonial legacies, neoliberal extractivism, and Eurocentric knowledge systems' prevailing views of disability discourse. The writer resorts to decolonial theory, indigenous knowledge systems, and the intersectional disability justice approaches to illustrate how coloniality has laid down the parameters of capability, productivity, and independence, which generally classify indigenous, afro-descendant, rural, queer, and disabled bodies as marginal. The chapter primarily emphasizes the indigenous views of interconnectedness, mutuality, and group care, thus showing that these cosmologies not only counter Western individualism but also present to society alternatives of justice that are based on land, community, and spirituality. Moreover, the chapter mentions the linkages with the struggles of the indigenous peoples for land, the environmental justice campaigns, and the neurodiversity and autistic activism in Brazil. It insinuates that the disability justice movement in Latin America is closely connected with the fight against racial capitalism, ecological destruction, and the oppression of knowledge. Simultaneously, it holds the universal human rights instruments accountable for their failures if they are not associated with local cultural contexts, thus advocating an interpretation that recognizes the multiple ontologies of disability. The disability justice project is perceived as one that is community-led, cross-cutting, and transformative; redefined by the interaction of the Global South, grassroots movement building, and the production of knowledge free from colonial influences. This chapter's emphasis on Global South experiences leads to the reshaping of disability studies into the more equitable, context-aware, and liberating futures still to come.

Keywords Decolonial disability justice · Latin America · Indigenous epistemologies · Intersectionality · And relationality

S. M. Thomas and R. Veerabathiran, *Disability and Decolonial Thought in Latin America*, SpringerBriefs in Modern Perspectives on Disability Research,
https://doi.org/10.1007/978-981-95-8950-0_6

6.1 Introduction

The disability justice movement in Latin America is more and more associated with decolonial thought, which is breaking through the traditional rights-based and biomedical frameworks that have always been unable to express the region's uniqueness in its history and social and cultural aspects (Ferrari, 2020; Lapierre, 2023). This new perspective illustrates that disability is not only an individual's impairment or a matter of legal rights, but it is also power relations that have had a substantial impact on Stigma and, therefore, on the exclusion of people with disabilities (Berthelot-Raffard, 2024; Ferrari, 2020; Lapierre, 2023).

Disability studies and interventions have mostly come from the Global North, which has resulted in a lack of recognition of the Global South's experiences. This China-centric view neglects the colonial and colonialism impacts that have not only disabled but also destructive for the native people and others in Latin America. Different factors have been creating "impaired peoples" through colonial legacies such as disadvantaged economic conditions, political violence, and environmental injustices (Gimenez, 2023; Grech, 2017; Lapierre, 2023; Meekosha, 2011). Decolonial thought is a powerful tool that helps one understand how this historical power relations still shape and are expressed in today's views and treatments of disability (Ferrari, 2020; Gandarilla Salgado et al., 2021; Grech, 2017).

Decolonial feminisms, for example, point to the coloniality of gender and its interaction with disability, asking for an ontological understanding of disability that contests the prevailing feminist and disability discourses (de Lima Costa, 2020; Mendoza & Grijalva, 2022). Marcela Beatriz Ferrari brings out the importance of decolonial feminism's analytical categories in the discourse about the definition of disability in the Latin American context, suggesting that decolonial thinking opens doors to the establishment of new analytical categories in social sciences at the intersection with disability issues (Ferrari, 2020). This view is in tune with the larger decolonial movement in Latin America, which has been questioning the modernity project and the still widespread European cultural imaginary as the root causes of social and environmental injustices (Rodríguez & Inturias, 2018; von Peter & Bieler, 2017).

The Convention on the Rights of Persons with Disabilities (CRPD) is a landmark international instrument that enshrines the human rights of persons with disabilities and gives a sociopolitical rather than a medical interpretation to disability (von Peter & Bieler, 2017).

On the other hand, even the rights-based approaches like the CRPD can be interpreted through a decolonial view, and then it would be guaranteed that the implementation respects and incorporates the various cultural perceptions of disability, particularly those from indigenous peoples. In fact, such people in Latin America often view and treat disability in terms of their cultural backgrounds, which are different from the prevailing notions of disability resulting from the historical oppression and forced cultural assimilation (Lapierre, 2023).

The idea of "coloniality of power" articulated by Aníbal Quijano is key to the re-definition of the issue (Gandarilla Salgado et al., 2021; Quijano, 2016; Taylor, 2016). Coloniality is not synonymous with colonialism, as it mainly focuses on the lasting power relations that were established during the colonial period and still exist in a modified form in the so-called post-colonial world, whereby they determine the nature of knowledge, power, and social relations (Gandarilla Salgado et al., 2021; Grech, 2017). This paradigm uncovers the fact that the categories of ability and disability are shaped in a certain way within these colonial structures of power (Berthelot-Raffard, 2024). To illustrate: academic ableism that exists in North American universities, although such institutions may have policies aimed at equity and inclusion, still largely neglects accessibility matters for persons with disabilities, indicating a more profound "capacitalism," which is unavoidably linked to the "intellectual contract" of universities built on colonial grounds 3. Consequently, it is very likely that even such well-meaning EDI (equity, diversity, and inclusion) programs may not be entirely successful if they do not confront the underlying coloniality that effectively determines who is "able" and who is not, thereby creating inequities (Berthelot-Raffard, 2024; Boda et al., 2022).

Exclusion against persons with disabilities in Latin America is not a mere question of individual bias or lack of accommodation, but rather a systemic problem supported by the colonial power structures (Berthelot-Raffard, 2024; Boda et al., 2022; Lapierre, 2023). For example, the coloniality of extractivism impacts environmental and territorial rights, with indigenous communities being the ones who suffer the most, among other factors, through disability (Gimenez, 2023; Hesketh, 2025; Losada Cubillos et al., 2023). This brings to light the need for an ecoterritorial turn in transitional and environmental justice talks that recognize the coloniality of nature (Kerremans & Destrooper, 2023; Losada Cubillos et al., 2023; Mollett, 2021; Rodriguez, 2020). Decolonial thought in Latin America, thus, aims at defeating these hegemonic systems by mapping out intellectual genealogies and practicing transgressive hermeneutics to reinterpret existing theories in their socio-historical and geopolitical contexts (Fúnez-Flores et al., 2022).

The decolonial strategy advocates a critical scrutiny of the way in which the prevailing narratives, mostly Eurocentric, fix the concepts of normalcy and pathology, thus rendering the other ways of being and knowing to be marginalized (Grech, 2017; Maniglio & Barboza da Silva, 2021). This implies not only the decolonization of knowledge production processes but also the comprehension of the subjective decoupling processes in the hegemonic groups like the medical professionals, which is a necessary step in the transformation of mental health systems in countries like Chile (Sepúlveda Jara & Oyarce Pisani, 2020). The objective is to arrive at a more inclusive interpretation of the concept of resilience, which is a step further from the current prescriptive, hegemonic, positivist, and ability-centric definitions that constrain disability studies (Hutcheon & Lashewicz, 2014).

In the end, reframing disability justice through a decolonial lens in Latin America means acknowledging that not only the whole spectrum of struggles of people with disabilities against colonialism, capitalism, and all kinds of oppressions are tightly connected (Berthelot-Raffard, 2024; Smith & Lester, 2023; Veillette, 2021).

It promotes the Global Southern self-determination, community-led initiatives, and epistemologies like "Bien Vivir," which can provide alternative social life frameworks outside the coloniality of power (Sonetti-González et al., 2023; da Silva et al., 2023, Quijano, 2016). It also means to accept the indigenous view, to oppose the racialized sexualities dictated by coloniality, and to apply the intersectional analysis that would reveal the hidden layers of injustice disabled people in the area are experiencing (Boda et al., 2022; Mollett, 2021; Schramm, 2012; Veillette, 2021). By way of example, the autistic activism in Brazil represents the movement that leads to neurodiversity and inalienable rights, aiming at the eradication of ableistic views and the promotion of social inclusion, which are among the essential elements of decolonial disability justice (da Nóbrega Rogoski et al., 2024).

6.2 Disability Justice in Latin America: Historical and Political Contexts

The historical and political contexts in Latin America have a significant influence on the disability justice movement, mainly the colonial legacies, the spread of neoliberalism, and the structural disablement that many people experience as a result of these policies (Lapierre, 2023; Meekosha, 2011; Rodríguez & Inturias, 2018). The interrelation of these factors has given rise to justice claims that are not only related to the dominant issues but also to the Indigenous, African-descendant, and peasant groups that are most affected by these systemic problems (Hesketh, 2025; Lapierre, 2023; Rodríguez & Inturias, 2018).

The legacies of colonization have created the fundamental factors that define disability and exclusion in terms of others all over Latin America (Ferrari, 2020; Lapierre, 2023; Meekosha, 2011). The Euro-American dominance in global disability discourse has consistently undermined the voices and views of the Global South, even being very reluctant to acknowledge that colonization itself was a disabling and killing process for the people living in these regions (Grech, 2017; Meekosha, 2011). This view, known as "coloniality of ability" or "coloniality of capacity," asserts that contemporary concepts of ability and disability are still determined by those very colonial power structures that classified and subjugated bodies according to racial, social, and economic criteria (Berthelot-Raffard, 2024; Ferrari, 2020). The idea of "coloniality of power" proposed by Aníbal Quijano is fundamental here, as it describes how the dynamics of domination set up during the colonial period still influence the production of knowledge, the organization of society, and the people's experiences of disability in post-colonial situations (Boda et al., 2022; Gandarilla Salgado et al., 2021). The coloniality that persists in today's world facilitates the operation of a system where certain bodies are labeled "able" and others "disabled" based on criteria that serve the interests of the hegemon, which are usually associated with profitability and the economic use of people under a capitalist system (Berthelot-Raffard, 2024; Boda et al., 2022).

The shift toward neoliberal economic policies in Latin America has made the problem of structural disablement even worse. Neoliberalism, which is mainly supported by the extractive industries, puts more pressure on natural resources and labor and often affects Indigenous and Afro-descendant areas and people the most. This "extractive logic of the coloniality of nature" makes the environmental degradation, forced displacement, and no access to vital services areas the production of disablement and impairment (Gimenez, 2023; Hesketh, 2025; Kerremans & Destrooper, 2023; Losada Cubillos et al., 2023). The case is given of mining in Brazil that, as in the past, the colonial rule continues to endanger the very existence and health of the native peoples, which influences their overall health negatively and increases the number of disabled people in such communities (Gimenez, 2023). The whole situation is the colonial power matrix that is combined with neoliberal extractivism, and that results in the social and environmental injustices in the first place. The mentioned injustices are mainly suffered by the poor and marginalized groups and thus can be regarded as structural disablement (Kerremans & Destrooper, 2023; Rodriguez, 2020; Rodríguez & Inturias, 2018). The massive number of environmental conflicts in Latin America, which are mostly connected with the development of neo-extractivism, mainly impacts the Indigenous people whose lands are pivotal for these activities (Hesketh, 2025).

The Indigenous, Afro-descendant, and peasant communities in Latin America have been the first to acknowledge the great injustices and have always been the ones who struggle for disability justice based on the traditional rights-based or biomedical frameworks; however, this is not the case now (Lapierre, 2023; Rodríguez & Inturias, 2018). To a large extent, their struggle is powered by the decolonial environmental justice approach, which asserts that social and ecological injustices, including those that cause disability, are products of modernity and the continuing spread of a European cultural imaginary (Rodríguez & Inturias, 2018; Rodríguez, 2020). Such movements place a significant focus on the decolonization of knowledge and social relations as the very crucial element that would lead to the lifting of historical oppression and marginalization (Rodríguez & Inturias, 2018).

By way of example, the native inhabitants view and treat disability from their very own perspectives and through their cultural practices, which at times go against the Western biomedical models (Lapierre, 2023). In fact, their fights for justice are often intertwined with land rights, cultural preservation, and self-determination, thereby acknowledging that their well-being, including the issue of disability, is tightly bound to their ancestral lands and traditional ways of living (da Nóbrega Rogoski et al., 2024). The idea of "ecoterritorial conflict resolution" and an "ecoterritorial turn in transformative transitional justice" are new concepts being introduced that highlight the strong connections between human rights, territorial integrity, and environmental justice, especially for indigenous and local people who are facing violence over the extraction of resources (Kerremans & Destrooper, 2023).

In the same manner, Afro-descendant and peasant communities find themselves in a position of structural disablement due to the historical discrimination, land dispossession, and systemic poverty imposed on them, all of which are compounded by the colonial and neoliberal forces. Their battles usually consist of fighting for access to health care, education, and job opportunities that are on a par with those of the majority, and at the same time, restoring their cultural identities and confronting the racialized structures that are responsible for their marginalization, vulnerability to impairment, and hence, poverty (Boda et al., 2022). The autistic activism movement in Brazil is an excellent example of contemporary community-led dialogues promoting neurodiversity and contesting ableist views in the region and is depicted in Fig. 6.1. Trying to achieve social inclusion and an intersectional view of autism, this movement, which has a daily aim to promote and defend the human rights of autistic individuals, is constantly dealing with the issues of diagnostic culture and biomedical perspectives. The movement's goal is to ensure that the rights of autistic individuals are recognized and upheld, reflecting a decolonial approach to disability justice that supports and includes, along with challenging the paradigms of power (da Nóbrega Rogoski et al., 2024).

The bloodshed actually highlights the need for a decolonial approach to disability rights in Latin America, which is able to spot and take apart the historical and present impacts of coloniality and neoliberalism so that there are accurate equity and inclusion for everyone, especially for those most marginalized (Ferrari, 2020;

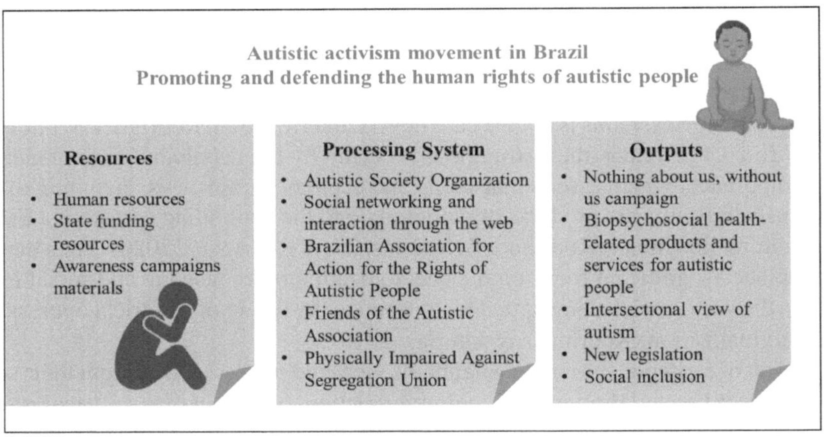

Fig. 6.1 Autistic activism movement in Brazil. The figure outlines the key components of the Brazilian autistic activism movement aimed at promoting and defending the human rights of autistic people. This figure presents a systems-based overview of autistic activism in Brazil, structured into Resources, Processing System, and Outputs. The Resources include human resources, state funding, and awareness campaign materials that support activism initiatives. The Processing System represents the organizational and social mechanisms driving the movement, including autistic-led organizations, web-based social networking and interaction, advocacy groups such as the Brazilian Association for Action for the Rights of Autistic People, allies' organizations, and disability rights unions opposing segregation. The Outputs highlight the outcomes of these collective efforts, including the "Nothing about us, without us" campaign, development of biopsychosocial health-related services and products, an intersectional understanding of autism, new legislation, and enhanced social inclusion. Thus, this figure illustrates how coordinated resources and advocacy structures translate into rights-based, inclusive outcomes for autistic people in Brazil

Rodríguez & Inturias, 2018; Rodríguez, 2020). Such an approach does not just mean giving the rights to the previously marginalized people who were left off from the existing rights frameworks, but requires reconfiguring the understanding of disability and justice fundamentally according to the different cultures and historical styles of Latin America (Ferrari, 2020; Rodríguez & Inturias, 2018).

6.3 Disability Justice and Indigenous Struggles

The indigenous views of justice, care, and interdependence related to disability in Latin America not only present a challenge to the Western paradigms but also underline the importance of relationality, reciprocity, and collective responsibility over individualistic auto and productive notions (Lapierre, 2023; Polheim et al., 2024). These indigenous systems of thought are based on worldviews that often stand in sharp contrast to the dominant medical and social models of disability that the Global North has (Lapierre, 2023; Meekosha, 2011).

In the indigenous people of Latin America, loyalty, reciprocity, and shared duty are the core values that shape the understanding and handling of disability (Lapierre, 2023). Instead of the Western fixation on the individual as completely independent and autonomous, many indigenous people see individuals as being very closely related to their families, communities, and the natural world (Okoliko, 2024; Polheim et al., 2024). Such a relational ontology implies that the well-being of everyone, including that of disabled people, is a collective concern and should not be placed entirely on the individual (Begay & Klor, 2024; Okoliko, 2024). For instance, relationality studies in the Ecuadorian Amazon point out that recognizing these interlinked relationships is critical for not only resolving sustainability issues but also human well-being issues in those communities. Thereby, in the case of disability, a system is created where care and support are rendered through a mutual network, stressing the duties and responsibilities of the community members rather than official help or individual rights (Polheim et al., 2024). This is the opposite of the Western notion of autonomy, which tends to characterize freedom as the absence of dependence on others, while a relational perspective holds that the very freedom lies in the relationships that enable.

The concept of indigenous disability in Latin America is often at odds with Western understanding of autonomy and productivity (Boda, 2022; Lapierre, 2023). Neoliberal performance criteria dictate that Western societies place the most importance on an individual's ability to work and economic contribution, which can lead to the exclusion of those with disabilities who do not conform to such standards (Brown & Leigh, 2018; Waterfield et al., 2018). Indigenous spirituality, on the other hand, does not necessarily grant individuals value based on their economic output. One can find disabled persons under the illuminating cultural practices and worldviews that accept and even highlight various kinds of contributions and belonging, stressing the person's innate quality within the group, irrespective of their productive capacity (Lapierre, 2023; Polheim et al., 2024). The debate about disability has been dominated by the Global North, resulting in these people's experiences being sidelined, thereby creating an "intellectual crisis for disability studies in the periphery" (Meekosha, 2011). The so-called intellectual imperialism has always imposed medicalized definitions of disability that ignore specific cultural understanding (Lapierre, 2023; Waterfield et al., 2018).

Disability justice is one of the concepts that serves as a link between disability and indigenous rights in Latin America (Boda, 2022; Payne-Tsoupros, 2020). The impact of colonialism on indigenous peoples has been immense; it has even produced disabilities as a result of historical and ongoing processes like colonization, forced assimilation, poverty, and political violence (Boda, 2022; Lapierre, 2023). The "disabling and devastating" consequences of colonization and colonialism in the Global South continue to generate populations with impairments (Meekosha, 2011). Thus, in these societies, being disabled is not simply a medical or individual concern but a situation deeply rooted in a history of systemic oppression and injustice (Boda, 2022; Lapierre, 2023). Disability justice, as a critical social theory, not only aligns with decolonial efforts but also goes along with the processes of identity-making that put forward the idea of the lives most valued and the rest less so because of the "racial capitalist coloniality." This perspective pushes for a murmuring that accepts the historical and structural determinants of disability suffered by indigenous groups (Boda, 2022).

Disability justice alliances with broader social justice movements in Latin America, including the feminist, queer, and decolonial ones (Boda, 2022; Deerinwater et al., 2024). The original Disability Justice Collective, which was made up of disabled queers of color, pointed out that the traditional disability rights movements were often overlooking the experiences of those with multiple marginalized identities (Deerinwater et al., 2024). In the case of Latin America, this intersectional approach is of utmost importance. Feminist and queer movements are in the for front advocating for the rights and the recognition of women and LGBTQ+ people, and when coupled with disability justice, they not only address the issue of predominantly marginalization faced by disabled women and queer men but also by the indigenous peoples (Deerinwater et al., 2024; González Villamizar & Bueno-Hansen, 2021; Snider, 2021; Stienstra, 2023). For example, incorporating intersectionality in contexts like the Truth Commission in Colombia has already been proven to bring about the exposure of "patriarchal, racialized and class-based structures of oppression" that restrict the complete participation of Indigenous and Afro-descendant women (González Villamizar & Bueno-Hansen, 2021).

Labor, migration, and disability precarity are massive challenges in Latin America, where disability justice is one of the main issues considered along with other social justice issues (Derakhshan & Chowdhury, 2025; Lapierre, 2023). The indigenous peoples usually live under deplorable social and economic conditions and are attacked by the government, among other causes of disabilities (Lapierre, 2023). Migration can make the situation of people very vulnerable, e.g., undocumented migrants who suffer from severe exploitation and isolation, and this in turn leads to "socio-economic immobility" and "systemic incapability." The difficulties disabled migrants face are further increased by not having access to social assistance, law courts, and even basic support (Derakhshan & Chowdhury, 2025). Their plight is primarily due to multiplicatively oppressive systems, which call for a disability justice approach that is intersectional.

In the struggle for disability rights, especially in Latin America, the concept of intersectionality is crucial (Amorim-Maia & Olazabal, 2024; Boda, 2022; González Villamizar & Bueno-Hansen, 2021). It states that social identities such as race, gender, class, and disability do not exist independently but instead overlap to produce wide and usually mixed discrimination and privilege experiences. Accordingly, it is not enough to speak about disability being one of the factors; instead, the dialogue must continue by pointing to the interrelations between the various social categories such as indigeneity, gender, race, and so on (Bixby, 2024; Boda, 2022; Saia et al., 2024). For instance, when it comes to the issue of deafness, it becomes apparent that the different disability groups or different age groups, and so on, have in common and what differentiates the social aspects of the problem (Bishop et al., 2024; Bixby, 2024).

An intersectional framework acknowledges the fact that a disabled indigenous woman residing in a remote area of Latin America experiences limitations that are entirely different from those of a non-disabled urban man, and therefore, activism needs to deal with these particular and interconnected kinds of oppression. This is shown by studies which indicate that "intersectional climate justice" needs to tackle gender and race inequalities in order to mitigate the causes of different vulnerabilities (Amorim-Maia & Olazabal, 2024).

The disability studies field is being asked to decolonize itself and, at the same time, to develop local adaptation strategies that would be appropriate to the local worldviews and that would even include the indigenous values and knowledge (Leal Filho et al., 2024; Meekosha, 2011). Acknowledging indigenous knowledge systems and moving away from Western-centric paradigms to more relational and culturally sensitive approaches are pivotal to the attainment of real disability justice in Latin America (Lapierre, 2023; Polheim et al., 2024; Riley et al., 2024).

6.4 Decolonizing Disability Justice in Latin America

The formation of alliances among diverse communities and movements is of utmost importance for the progress of decolonial disability justice in Latin America, which involves the coming together of Indigenous, disabled, and other disadvantaged groups (Boda, 2022; Lapierre, 2023; Meekosha, 2011). The process typically requires the use of grassroots organizing, mutual aid, and community care practices, which are totally at odds with the individualistic Western way of thinking about disability (Meekosha, 2011; Polheim et al., 2024). In addition to that, transnational solidarities and South–South dialogues play a crucial role in the development of a united, decolonial answer to the problems of disability, which not only go beyond geographic boundaries but also encompass shared colonial histories (Boda, 2022; Meekosha, 2011).

The collaboration of Indigenous, disabled, and marginalized groups is a prerequisite for the proper handling of the complex, intersectional nature of disability in Latin America (Boda, 2022; Lapierre, 2023). The occurrence of disability among the indigenous people of Latin America is high, and the phenomenon is influenced by their particular worldviews, cultural practices, and the continuance of colonialism, forced assimilation, and socio-economic inequalities that are otherwise characterized as the main barriers to their development (Lapierre, 2023). The Global South's experience with colonialism has been both disabling and devastating, and it continues to do so by producing impaired populations as a result of various phenomena (Meekosha, 2011). That is why the building of unity between these groups accepts that disability is not exclusively a medical matter but is closely linked to historical oppression, systemic inequalities, and the contests for self-determination (Boda, 2022; Lapierre, 2023; Meekosha, 2011). It will then be through these coalitions that a more inclusive perspective on disability will emerge, seeing it as a consequence of "racial capitalist coloniality," where certain lives are rendered less valuable according to their simultaneous identities (Boda, 2022).

The grassroots organizing, mutual aid, and community care practices represent not only the ultimate means of support but the Indigenous perception of justice, care, and interdependence. While Western models often rely on formal services and institutional support, most Indigenous communities give priority to relationality, reciprocity, and collectivism. As a result, disabled people's care is seamlessly integrated into the networks of the community, where well-being is a collective duty instead of a personal burden (Polheim et al., 2024). This way of thinking is in direct opposition to the Western ideas of independence and efficiency, which often leave aside those who do not meet the market standards of contribution. Instead, it is considered through the lens of a person's inherent value in the community, regardless of their ability to be productive (Lapierre, 2023). The nurturing and political attitudes of care development are one of the main parts of the community-centric strategies, which correspond with the intersectional climate justice frameworks focusing on social equity (Amorim-Maia & Olazabal, 2024).

Coalitions between different nations and dialogues between Southern countries are the two most important factors to provide a solid base for disability rights in decolonialism. The North's power in the disability conversation has made the Global South's experiences less heard, creating an "intellectual crisis for disability studies in the periphery." The talks between South and South promote the sharing of knowledge, the adoption of strategies, and the strengthening of ties among the communities that were once under colonial rule, thus empowering them to fight against the Western disability concept that claims to be universal. This is especially true considering that a large number of the countries in the South have the same colonial past, which has a significant impact on their disability experience (Boda, 2022; Meekosha, 2011).

Moreover, arts, knowledge making, and political vision are among the most effective decolonial disability justice enablers in the Latin American region. More than that, storytelling, memory, and physical resistance, to name just a few, are indispensable in putting back in the center the narratives of those who have been neglected and in disputing the usual portrayals of disabled people. In fact, Native peoples, for example, do not just tell their stories to be recognized, but to prove that there is a connection between what happened in the past and today's society, and to present colonial archival practices that are often contextless as one of the problem areas. These expressive forms give an opportunity to disabled people and Native communities to share their stories, to claim their identity, and to recover their past outside the Western systems (Begay & Klor, 2024; Lapierre, 2023). Such methods are in line with the idea of "weaving stories of strength," which is the basis for including Indigenous viewpoints into larger educational and professional development programs (Riley et al., 2024).

Decolonizing disability knowledge and representation in Latin America is a process that means critically dissecting and tearing apart the Western-centric biases that are already in the field of disability studies and practices. The intellectual decolonization in this case would be aiming at replacing the universalizing narratives with the context-specific ones that are culturally informed and have the characteristics of the various realities of the Latin American populations (Meekosha, 2011). Besides that, it also means confronting the concealed "identity-making" processes that are a part of "racial capitalist coloniality" and through which certain lives are made to appear more valuable than others (Boda, 2022). By lifting Indigenous knowledge systems and relating worldviews, decoupling intends to create a new environment for knowledge generation that would not only be beneficial to the local communities in terms of empowerment but also facilitate and support self-determined approaches to disability (Begay & Klor, 2024; Lapierre, 2023; Polheim et al., 2024).

Notwithstanding the aforementioned efforts, however, difficulties and contradictions remain regarding the decolonial disability justice in Latin America. The presence of internal hierarchies, exclusion, and co-optation can act as a deterrent to solidarity movements. It is the very same power imbalances that may prevail in the case of marginalized communities that will lead to the exclusion of some voices, thus reproducing the pattern of exclusion. The Disability Justice Collective, for example, came into being as a response to the way in which the mainstream Disability Rights Movement had practically ignored the experiences of disabled queers of color, thus pointing to the very necessity of not only being but also continuously checking and challenging internal hierarchies (Deerinwater et al., 2024). These divisions within the movement can not only render the coalition-building less effective and dilute the power of collective action (Saia et al., 2024).

Negotiating state recognition and autonomy alongside still other significant obstacles. On one hand, the gain of state recognition translates into the availability of resources and legal safeguards; on the other hand, the risk of co-optation is also present, whereby Indigenous and disability movements might get forced into the conforming circle of state-defined categories and priorities that are contrary to their decolonial goals. The dilemma was not an easy one because it was about balancing the positive aspects of state structures' engagement with the possible negative aspects of autonomy and self-determination erosion. In most cases, the issue involved navigating complex political landscapes where disability was linked with the larger issues of land rights, cultural preservation, and political sovereignty. This is an even bigger challenge for women and girls with disabilities, as they are the most marginalized group and are protected by rights that are full of loopholes, leading to their lack of access to education, health, public services, and justice. In fact, to tackle these issues, it is necessary to use an intersectional approach that takes into account disability as a significant factor of stratification in sociological research (Bixby, 2024; Lapierre, 2023; Meekosha, 2011; Stienstra, 2023).

The ongoing issues underscore the necessity of constant critical reflection and adaptive strategies, which are to become the hallmarks of the decolonial disability justice movements in Latin America. It is the complicated interaction of colonial legacies, socio-economic factors, and different cultural interpretations of disability that calls for a very subtle and much localized approach, at the same time being able to unite broader solidarities.

6.5 Toward Transformative Futures: Reimagining Policy, Activism, and Praxis

Moving "Toward Transformative Futures" for disability in Latin America means a total policy, activism, and praxis reimagination along with disability justice, which is a collective, decolonial project as the foundation. This approach goes beyond just integrating disability with the existing structures to seriously questioning and even reshaping them to cater to the historical and systemic marginalization that disabled individuals, especially those from the Indigenous and other marginalized communities, have gone through.

Reimagining policy, activism, and praxis in Latin America demands a critical review of the traditional understanding and response to disability issues. The North's dominance in global disability discourse has, in the past, led to the neglect of the civil rights and social justice experiences from the South, thus creating an "intellectual crisis for disability studies in the periphery" (Meekosha, 2011). Hence, the need for policies to move away from the universalizing, often Western-centric models to those that are culturally informed and context-specific, which will be able to capture the diverse realities of Latin American populations (Lapierre, 2023). Not only that, but also the integration of Indigenous epistemologies and relational worldviews into policy frameworks, which prioritize collective well-being and interdependence over individualistic notions of autonomy and productivity (Meekosha, 2011). Therefore, activism must go beyond the typical disability rights fight, which has sometimes ignored the intersecting oppressions faced by disabled queer people of color, for example, to take up a broader disability justice framework (Deerinwater et al., 2024). The taking of theory into practice, or praxis, must therefore be a vehicle for these remade policies and the resilient forms of dissent they have stirred up, thereby introducing and rooting in local and conventional practices the likes of grassroots organizing, mutual aid, and community care (Lapierre, 2023).

In this light, disability justice is a communal, decolonial undertaking (Boda, 2022). It recognizes that in Latin America, disability is not merely a medical issue but rather a socio-economic and political condition very much tied to colonialism, forced assimilation, and violence (Lapierre, 2023). The process of colonization has been "both disabling and devastating" for the Global South, thus constantly giving rise to populations with impaired abilities (Meekosha, 2011). Hence, a decolonial disability justice project will seek to wipe out the "racial capitalist coloniality," allowing certain lives to be considered more valuable than others and thus denying the lives of Indigenous peoples the right to exist. This will require fighting against the identity-forming processes that the hierarchies rely on (Boda, 2022). The Disabled Rights Movements, consisting of Black and Brown disabled queer people, purposely turned a deaf ear to the fact that the main disability rights movements had practically forgotten the experiences of people with intersecting marginalized identities (Deerinwater et al., 2024). Henceforth, this indicates the necessity for disability justice to be an intrinsically intersectional project that collaborates with broader movements for social justice, such as feminist, queer, and decolonial movements (Snider, 2021). Such alliances recognize that the battles against sexism, racism, and economic oppression are inextricably linked to the struggle for disability justice, which is particularly true for women and girls with disabilities who are the most affected by systemic marginalization and lack of rights protection (Stienstra, 2023). By foregrounding the experiences and leadership of those at the intersections of multiple marginalized identities, disability justice as a decolonial project aims to foster genuine social transformation and equity (González Villamizar & Bueno-Hansen, 2021).

6.6 Conclusion

To us, the decolonial politics of disability justice in Latin America are not simply the expansion of the current disability rights frameworks but the complete rethinking of the concepts of disability, justice, and even humanity. This chapter shows that the history of disabilities in the area is so tightly interwoven with colonization, land theft, racialization, and neoliberalism that the latter have inflicted impairment and exclusion as a result. The theme of disability justice thus entails the confronting of power coloniality that discloses the value of lives, productivity of bodies, and legitimacy of knowledge. We suggest that Native American and community-based worldviews offer crucial routes toward the future of transformation. Their focus on the connections, interdependence, and shared accountability refutes the very values of autonomy, efficiency, and market that are installed in the Western models. Disability justice is, therefore, based on these perspectives, inseparable from environmental, gender, and cultural-justice struggles for sovereignty over lands and peoples. Notably, this kind of intervention fights against the unification of disability experiences and instead takes intersectionality as an essential methodological and political tool. Nonetheless, decolonial disability justice should always be self-reflective. The internal hierarchies, state co-optation risks, and the exclusions among movements can all lead to the same inequalities that the movements aim to abolish being reproduced. Absolutely, no doubt, permanent critical engagement, grassroots leadership, and getting the most marginalized, especially Indigenous women, queer, and multiply disabled persons, becoming the priority are the things that are very necessary. We, however, argue that disability justice in Latin America should be viewed as a living, collective praxis: one that mixes activism, care, storytelling, and policy changes to fight against colonial legacies and to envision dignified, plural, and self-determined ways of being.

References

Amorim-Maia, A. T., & Olazabal, M. (2024). Localising the Global Goal on Adaptation through intersectional thinking. *Cities, 154*, Article 105349. https://doi.org/10.1016/j.cities.2024.105349

Begay, V., & Klor, K. M. (2024). Provenance through storytelling: Application of indigenous relationality toward arrangement and description. *Archival Science, 24*(4), 611–635. https://doi.org/10.1007/s10502-024-09451-z

Berthelot-Raffard, A. (2024). From capacitalism to disability justice in academia: A philosophical manifesto. *Equity in Education & Society*. https://doi.org/10.1177/27526461241307326

Bishop, G. M., Llewellyn, G., Kavanagh, A. M., Badland, H., Bailie, J., Stancliffe, R., Emerson, E., Fortune, N., & Aitken, Z. (2024). Disability-related inequalities in the prevalence of loneliness across the lifespan: trends from Australia, 2003 to 2020. *BMC Public Health, 24*(1), 621. https://doi.org/10.1186/s12889-024-17936-w

Bixby, L. E. (2024). Intersectional inequalities: How socioeconomic well-being varies at the intersection of disability, gender, race-ethnicity, and age. *Research in Social Stratification and Mobility, 91*, Article 100938. https://doi.org/10.1016/j.rssm.2024.100938

Boda, P. A. (2022). Identity making as a colonization process, and the power of disability justice to cultivate intersectional disobedience. *Education Sciences, 12*(7), 462. https://doi.org/10.3390/educsci12070462

Boda, P. A., Nusbaum, E. A., & Kulkarni, S. S. (2022). From 'what is' toward 'what if'through intersectionality: Problematizing ableist erasures and coloniality in racially just research. *International Journal of Research & Method in Education, 45*(4), 356–369. https://doi.org/10.1080/1743727X.2022.2054981

Brown, N., & Leigh, J. (2018). Ableism in academia: Where are the disabled and ill academics? *Disability & Society, 33*(6), 985–989. https://doi.org/10.1080/09687599.2018.1455627

da Nóbrega Rogoski, B., Caldas, R. C. S., Souza Guevara, V. L. D., Louzeiro, R., Vasconcelos, L. A., & Flores, E. P. (2024). Autism activism movement in Brazil: Contingency analysis and the Pacto pela Neurodiversidade (Pledge for Neurodiversity). *Trends in Psychology*, 1–20. https://doi.org/10.1007/s43076-024-00406-y

da Silva, R. F., Torres-Rivera, A. D., Pereira, V. A., Cardoso, L. R., & Becerra, M. J. (2023). Critical environmental education in Latin America from a socio-environmental perspective: Identity, territory, and social innovation. *Sustainability, 15*(12), 9410. https://doi.org/10.3390/su15129410

de Lima Costa, C. (2020). Latin America, decoloniality, and translation: Feminists building connectant epistemologies. https://doi.org/10.1093/oso/9780190062965.003.0011

Deerinwater, J., Ho, S., Thompson, V., Wong, A., Erevelles, N., & Morrow, M. (2024). A conversation on disability justice and intersectionality. In *Handbook of disability: Critical thought and social change in a globalizing world* (pp. 503–524). Springer Nature Singapore.

Derakhshan, R., & Chowdhury, R. (2025). Experience of marginalization in noncooperative spaces: The case of undocumented migrant workers in Italy. *Journal of Business Ethics, 197*(2), 231–252. https://doi.org/10.1007/s10551-024-05749-1

Ferrari, M. B. (2020). Feminismos descoloniales y discapacidad: hacia una conceptualización de la colonialidad de la capacidad. *Nómadas,* (52), 115–131. https://doi.org/10.30578/nomadas.n52a7

Fúnez-Flores, J. I., Díaz Beltrán, A. C., & Jupp, J. (2022). Decolonial discourses and practices: Geopolitical contexts, intellectual genealogies, and situated pedagogies. *Educational Studies, 58*(5–6), 596–619. https://doi.org/10.1080/00131946.2022.2132393

Gandarilla Salgado, J. G., García-Bravo, M. H., & Benzi, D. (2021). Two decades of Anibal Quijano's coloniality of power, Eurocentrism and Latin America. *Contexto Internacional, 43,* 199–222. https://doi.org/10.1590/s0102-8529.2019430100009

Gimenez, R. B. M. (2023). The Pandemic's Golden Touch: (Neo) Extractivism, Coloniality, and Necropolitics on Brazil's Indigenous Territories. *Canadian Journal of Law and Society/la Revue Canadienne Droit Et Société, 38*(3), 352–371. https://doi.org/10.1017/cls.2023.28

González Villamizar, J., & Bueno-Hansen, P. (2021). The promise and perils of mainstreaming intersectionality in the Colombian peace process. *International Journal of Transitional Justice, 15*(3), 553–575. https://doi.org/10.1093/IJTJ/IJAB026

Grech, S. (2017). Decolonising Eurocentric disability studies: Why colonialism matters in the disability and global South debate. In *Disability and colonialism* (pp. 6–21). Routledge. https://doi.org/10.1080/13504630.2014.995347

Hesketh, C. (2025). Indigenous resistance at the frontiers of accumulation: Challenging the coloniality of space in international relations. *Review of International Studies, 51*(1), 64–83. https://doi.org/10.1017/S0260210523000268

Hutcheon, E., & Lashewicz, B. (2014). Theorizing resilience: Critiquing and unbounding a marginalizing concept. *Disability & Society, 29*(9), 1383–1397. https://doi.org/10.1080/09687599.2014.934954

Kerremans, S., & Destrooper, T. (2023). Exploring the nexus between transitional justice and ecoterritorial conflict resolution: Time for an ecoterritorial turn in transformative transitional justice? *International Journal of Transitional Justice, 17*(1), 54–70. https://doi.org/10.1093/ijtj/ijac026

Lapierre, M. (2023). Disability and Latin American indigenous peoples. *Disability & Society, 38*(7), 1276–1280. https://doi.org/10.1080/09687599.2023.2192381

Leal Filho, W., Luetz, J. M., Nunn, P. D., Turagabeci, A., & Campbell, D. (2024). Effective domestic climate policies to protect small island states. *Nature Climate Change, 14*(7), 660–661. https://doi.org/10.1038/s41558-024-02005-2

Losada Cubillos, J. J., Trujillo Quintero, H. F., & Lugo Perea, L. J. (2023). Extractive logic of the coloniality of nature: Feeling-thinking through agroecology as a decolonial project. *Capitalism Nature Socialism, 34*(1), 88–106. https://doi.org/10.1080/10455752.2022.2127416

Maniglio, F., & Barboza da Silva, R. (2021). El Análisis Crítico del Discurso y el giro decolonial¿ Por qué y para qué? *Critical Discourse Studies, 18*(1), 156–184. https://doi.org/10.1080/17405904.2020.1754871

Meekosha, H. (2011). Decolonising disability: Thinking and acting globally. *Disability & Society, 26*(6), 667–682. https://doi.org/10.1080/09687599.2011.602860

Mendoza, B., & Grijalva, D. P. (2022). The epistemology of the south, coloniality of gender, and Latin American Feminism. *Hypatia, 37*(3), 510–522. https://doi.org/10.1017/hyp.2022.26

Mollett, S. (2021). Hemispheric, relational, and intersectional political ecologies of race: Centring land-body entanglements in the Americas. *Antipode, 53*(3), 810–830. https://doi.org/10.1111/anti.12696

Okoliko, D. A. (2024). Reflecting on care within an African relational framework for environmental communication. *Environmental Communication, 18*(1–2), 8–14. https://doi.org/10.1080/17524032.2023.2296829

Payne-Tsoupros, C. (2020). A starting point for disability justice in Legal Education. *Journal Committed to Social Change on Race and Ethnicity (JCSCORE), 6*(1), 165–189. https://doi.org/10.15763/issn.2642-2387.2020.6.1.164-189

Polheim, A., Manuel-Navarrete, D., Goebel, J., & Loos, J. (2024). Embodying relationality through immersive sustainability solutions with Indigenous communities in the Ecuadorian Amazon. *Sustainability Science, 19*(4), 1445–1457. https://doi.org/10.1007/s11625-024-01523-4

Quijano, A. (2016). 'Bien Vivir'–Between 'Development'and the De/coloniality of Power. *Alternautas (Re) Searching Development: The Abya Yala Chapter, 3*(1), 10–23. https://doi.org/10.31273/alternautas.v3i1.1023

Riley, T., Meston, T., Cutler, C., Low-Choy, S., McCormack, B. A., Kim, E. J. A., Nakar, S., & Vasco, D. (2024). Weaving stories of strength: Ethically integrating Indigenous content in teacher education and professional development programmes. *Teaching and Teacher Education, 142*, 104513. https://doi.org/10.1016/j.tate.2024.104513

Rodriguez, I. (2020). Latin American decolonial environmental justice. In *Environmental justice* (pp. 78–93). Routledge. https://doi.org/10.4324/9780429029585-8

Rodríguez, I., & Inturias, M. L. (2018). Conflict transformation in indigenous peoples' territories: Doing environmental justice with a 'decolonial turn.' *Development Studies Research, 5*(1), 90–105. https://doi.org/10.1080/21665095.2018.1486220

Saia, T., Yaghmaian, R., Cuesta, R., Mueller, C., & Pebdani, R. N. (2024). A call to action for disability and rehabilitation research using a DisCrit and disability justice framework. *Disability and Rehabilitation, 46*(14), 3189–3195. https://doi.org/10.1080/09638288.2023.2242780

Schramm, C. (2012). Queering Latin American coloniality and the cross-cultural production of racialised sexualities. *Journal of Intercultural Studies, 33*(3), 347–362.

Sepúlveda Jara, R., & Oyarce Pisani, A. M. (2020). New and old knowledge aimed at decolonising mental health: Reflections and proposals from Chile. *International Review of Psychiatry, 32*(4), 334–339. https://doi.org/10.1080/09540261.2020.1767042

Smith, M. N., & Lester, C. A. (2023). From "dependency" to "decoloniality"? The enduring relevance of materialist political economy and the problems of a "decolonial" alternative. *Social Dynamics, 49*(2), 196–219. https://doi.org/10.1080/02533952.2023.2220588

Snider, S. (2021). Moving toward disability justice: Introduction to "lesbian lives, disabled lives." *Journal of Lesbian Studies, 25*(3), 159–162. https://doi.org/10.1080/10894160.2020.1778853

Sonetti-González, T., Mancilla García, M., Tengö, M., Tourne, D. C., De Castro, F., & Futemma, C. R. (2023). Foregrounding Amazonian women through decolonial and process-relational perspectives for transdisciplinary transformation. *Ecosystems and People, 19*(1), 2260503. https://doi.org/10.1080/26395916.2023.2260503

Stienstra, D. (2023). (Th) reading rights and justice: Women and girls with disabilities. *Global Society, 37*(3), 354–374. https://doi.org/10.1080/13600826.2022.2146576

Taylor, L. (2016). Decolonizing citizenship: Reflections on the coloniality of power in Argentina. In *Narratives and imaginings of citizenship in Latin America* (pp. 72–86). Routledge. https://doi.org/10.1080/13621025.2013.818375

Veillette, A. M. (2021). Racialized popular feminism: A decolonial analysis of women's struggle with police violence in Rio de Janeiro's favelas. *Latin American Perspectives, 48*(4), 87–104. https://doi.org/10.1177/0094582X211015324

von Peter, S., & Bieler, P. (2017). How to study chronic diseases—Implications of the convention on the rights of persons with disabilities for research designs. *Frontiers in Public Health, 5*, 88. https://doi.org/10.3389/fpubh.2017.00088

Waterfield, B., Beagan, B. B., & Weinberg, M. (2018). Disabled academics: A case study in Canadian universities. *Disability & Society, 33*(3), 327–348. https://doi.org/10.1080/09687599.2017.1411251

Chapter 7
Rethinking Inclusion, Rights, and Policy from the Grassroots

Abstract This chapter takes a critical look at disability inclusion, rights, and policy in Latin America by placing grassroots movements, Indigenous knowledge systems, and the lived experiences of disabled communities at the center. It challenges Western, rights-based, and institutional models that are dominant and argues that top-down approaches based on universalism, individualism, and legalism often do not manage to cope with the region's historically situated realities, which were shaped by colonialism, racial capitalism, forced assimilation, and political violence. Although international frameworks, such as the Convention on the Rights of Persons with Disabilities (CRPD), have expanded the scope of formal legal recognition, there remains a significant gap between rights on paper and justice in practice. By using decolonial disability studies, the chapter shows that disability is both produced and experienced relationally–it is closely tied to land dispossession, poverty, gendered violence, environmental injustice, and Indigenous marginalization. Grassroots and community-led movements are seen as central sites of policy knowledge, able to express alternative visions of inclusion grounded in relationality, reciprocity, collective care, and belonging rather than autonomy and productivity. The chapter is examining the issues of Indigenous self-governance, legal pluralism, participatory praxis, and pluriversal policy frameworks, and it is pointing out the existence of pathways toward disability justice that resist assimilation and co-optation. It also discusses ethical tensions such as the internal exclusions within movements and the risks of tokenistic state recognition. Finally, the chapter urges a shift from institutional access to lived justice–one that places self-determination, community-defined priorities, and South–South dialogues at the center. This chapter focuses on the bottom-up approach to envisioning inclusion in the first place, thereby playing a role in the formation of disability policies that are in tune with the culture, adapted to the place, and able to bring transformation in Latin America.

Keywords Legal pluralism · Decolonization · disability policy · Latin America · Pluriversality

S. M. Thomas and R. Veerabathiran, *Disability and Decolonial Thought in Latin America*, SpringerBriefs in Modern Perspectives on Disability Research,
https://doi.org/10.1007/978-981-95-8950-0_7

7.1 Introduction

The rethinking of Latin America's disability inclusion "from below" requires a very big change in the treatment of the disabled community, from passive to active acknowledgment of their experiences and recognizing the fights of the grassroots as the indispensable sites of policy knowledge. This method deeply opposes the classical top-down inclusion models that, most of the time, are rooted in Western perspectives and do not cater for the specific realities and historical contexts of disabled people in Latin America (Meekosha, 2011).

The changeover from the institutional to the lived notion of disability inclusion in Latin America means the pulling down of the barriers caused by policy and legislation, and putting the focus on the real lives of the disabled people. Institutional inclusion sought to make a place for people with disabilities in society by including them through high-standard methods. In contrast, lived inclusion regarded the qualitative factors of participation, belonging, and well-being within local cultural and socio-economic contexts as the most important (Lapierre, 2023). The Global North's control over the disability discourse has meant that the Global South's voices have been obscured, leading to an "intellectual crisis for disability studies in the periphery" (Meekosha, 2011). Consequently, the universalizing policies do not reflect the diverse needs, such as the ones that arose from colonialism, forced assimilation, and political violence, of Latin American indigenous peoples with disabilities that are thus highly affected in the first place (Lapierre, 2023). Hence, understanding lived inclusion necessitates policies that are not only culturally informed but also context-specific, recognizing the diverse realities and integrating indigenous epistemologies and relational worldviews that prioritize collective welfare and interdependence (Lapierre, 2023; Polheim et al., 2024). One part of the application of disability justice is to see suffering due to disability as interconnected with other factors and to treat it socially.

To put it another way, the movements in the grassroots are the first places where one can learn about policies in many parts of Latin America, when they show not only different but sometimes even totally unseen by institutional approaches, views, and solutions. This kind of activism is the result of the direct contact of the disadvantaged communities with the problems and thus is their very close understanding of their needs, cultural practices, and historical injustices (Lapierre, 2023). Thus, for instance, the indigenous peoples hardly ever fail to relate disability to their own worldviews and cultural practices, which may embrace aspects like relationality, reciprocity, and collective responsibility—absolutely contradicting the Western concepts of autonomy and productivity (Lapierre, 2023; Polheim et al., 2024; Bixby, 2024). The "Disability Justice Collective," consisting of disabled queer people of color, specifically pointed out that one of its goals was to appeal mainstream Disability Rights Movements that had practically turned a blind eye to the suffering of those with facing marginalized identities developing thus highlighting the pivotal role of grassroots movements in the production of inclusive policy knowledge (Deerinwater et al., 2024). These movements are now beginning to define the ethics and politics of care, place-based approaches, climate action and community resilience, and, importantly, the holistic view of justice that tackles gender and race inequalities and reduces the causes of differential vulnerabilities is not only signified but also recognized through their actions (Amorim-Maia & Olazabal, 2024).

The historical backdrop of colonialism has still immensely influenced the way disability was and is viewed in Latin America; thus, decoloniality in acceptance is a necessity. The colonial project, both "disabling and disastrous" to the people of the Global South, generated an impaired population through several processes (Meekosha, 2011). As a matter of fact, recognition of disability in Latin America is inseparable from acknowledging its ties with the colonialism legacies, forced assimilation, socio-economic disparity, and political violence (Lapierre, 2023). Movements from the ground up provide a strong counter-narrative to "racial capitalist coloniality" that undermines the worth of certain lives and experiences, among which the disability of the indigenous is included (Boda, 2022). Taking into account local knowledge and community solidarity, these contests lead to the development of more equitable, culturally relevant, and responsive policies that meet the complex needs of diverse communities. This policy knowledge that emerges from the bottom is also a support to the "weaving stories of strength" project, which ethically embeds Indigenous content into school curricula, thereby highlighting the role of real experiences in building effective policies and practices (Riley et al., 2024). It is the participation of diverse voices at the bottom that ensures that policies not only address systemic marginalization but also bring about real social change, as they do not reinforce existing power structures (Stienstra, 2023).

7.2 The Genealogy of Rights-Based Frameworks in Disability Policy

The history of rights-based frameworks in disability policy in Latin America can be traced back to principles of universalism, individualism, and legalism that came from the Global North liberalism. This has frequently led to the mere exporting of rights without the necessary local adaptation, causing difficulties in the application of policies that really meet the specific conditions of the region's disabled communities. This different frameworks of genealogy in disability policy are depicted in Fig. 7.1.

Universalism, individualism, and legalism are fundamental principles of this inherited framework. Universalism claims that certain rights and benefits are granted to every human being purely because they are human, no matter what the situation is. This argument could be called a "double-edged sword" as it will bring some advantages. However, at the same time, it will completely ignore the specific cultural, social, and economic factors that determine the disability in different places, for instance, Latin American Indigenous communities. Individualism considers the disabled person as the only one entitled to rights and often encourages the development of individual accommodations instead of the systemic changes that are rooted in the well-being of the whole community and the support from the community,

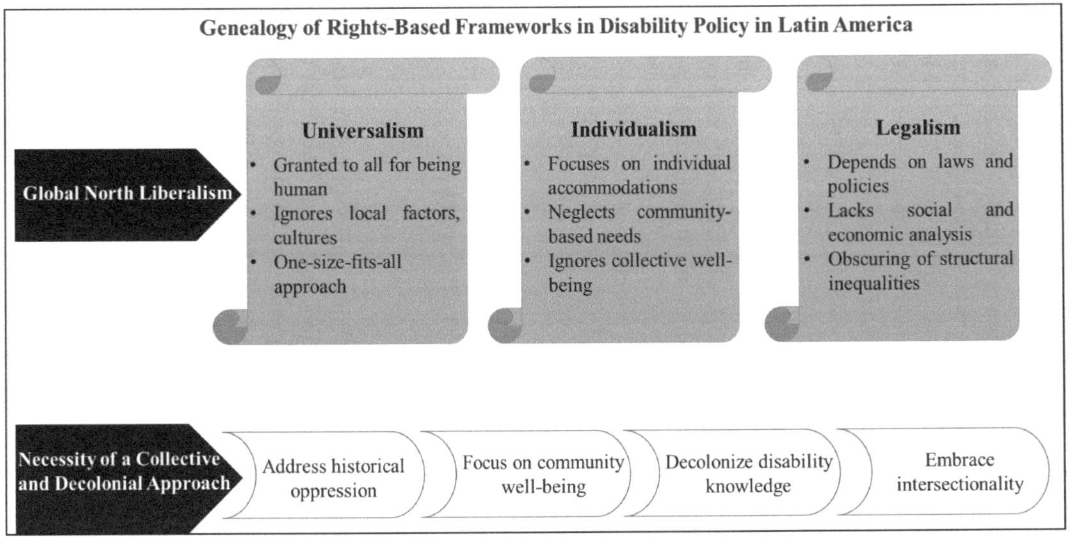

Fig. 7.1 Genealogy of rights-based frameworks in disability policy in Latin America. The figure traces dominant rights-based approaches shaping disability policy, highlighting their origins in Global North liberalism and the need for alternative frameworks. This figure illustrates the conceptual genealogy of rights-based disability policy frameworks influential in Latin America, rooted primarily in Global North liberalism. Three dominant paradigms are depicted: Universalism, which frames rights as inherent to all humans but often adopts a one-size-fits-all approach that overlooks local cultures and contexts; Individualism, which prioritizes individualized accommodations while neglecting community-based needs and collective well-being; and Legalism, which relies heavily on laws and policies but frequently lacks social and economic analysis and obscures structural inequalities. The lower section of the figure emphasizes the necessity of a collective and decolonial approach, calling for disability policies that move beyond individualistic and legalistic models to address historical, cultural, and structural realities in Latin America

which are three of the characteristics belonging to many Indigenous worldviews (Lapierre, 2023). Legalism considers legal and policy instruments as the primary channel to drive inclusion, often through formal recognition and anti-discrimination laws. While legal frameworks are undeniably important, over-dependence on them without dealing with the social, economic, and historical injustices can lead to insubstantial changes that do not actually affect the lives of the people involved. For instance, women and girls with disabilities are still victims of systematic marginalization and a lack of rights protections, which restrict their access to education, health, public services, and justice, even though there are legal provisions that exist (Stienstra, 2023).

The framework in question tends to export rights to Latin America without any reference to the local situation. The North, which is liberal in its policies, is latterly and very often prejudicially accepted in Latin America without proper modification for local conditions (Meekosha, 2011). This practice may prove to be very controversial, especially considering the history of the region, which has had a significant impact on the people and thus has given it a very different perception of disabled people (Lapierre, 2023). Colonialism's "disabling and devastating" effects still disallow population growth and thus continue to create impaired ones (Meekosha, 2011). When rights are granted, ignoring all these historical and structural factors, they may not coincide with the local views on disability, justice, and community. For example, the Indigenous groups in Latin America often see disability from their own perspectives, which emphasize interconnectedness, giving and taking, and collective accountability, whereas the Western viewpoint is very much individualistic and thus considers autonomy and productivity as the main facets of disability (Lapierre, 2023). Policies that do not take into consideration these cultural differences may not work at all or even worsen the present states of marginalization. This calls for decolonizing disability knowledge and representation, which means giving up universalizing narratives in favor of context-specific, culturally informed understandings (Meekosha, 2011).

The argument regarding the contradiction between the global rights frameworks and local realities emphatically highlights the necessity of a transition to a collective and decolonial approach of disability justice (Boda, 2022). It is therefore the case that the concept of disability has to be reshaped as not just a medical or individual matter but rather as a highly complex phenomenon that has a lot to do with the historical oppression and systematic inequalities and the fights for the right to self-determination (Boda, 2022; Lapierre, 2023). The merging of Indigenous ways of knowing and being that are the basis for policy frameworks, which give priority to the well-being of communities, is vital for the absolute acceptance of all (Lapierre, 2023). Besides, an intersectionality viewpoint is fundamental to analyze the disability as it overlaps with the other identities such as gender, race-ethnicity, and age, which lead to the creation of multiple layers of the inequality experience (Bixby, 2024). This thorough comprehension may help the policy to go beyond the formal rights declarations and to create the relevant and transformative lives for disabled people in Latin America, the inclusive lives that are actually experienced (Meekosha, 2011).

7.3 Formal Rights to Lived Justice: Power, Relationality, and Community Praxis

Although Western rights-based approaches to disability in Latin America, intending to achieve inclusive and equal societies, still face a lot of limitations that are mainly based on the region's historical, social, and political contexts (Taylor, 2016). The official legal acknowledgment of disability rights very often does not bring about any significant changes regarding the quality of life of disabled people and consequently creates a constant gap between what is legally accepted and the actual situation (Meléndez Rojas, 2019; Martínez Espinoza, 2015). Among the factors that cause this situation, the most significant are the bureaucracy involved, the lack of proper accessibility, the overall exclusion of people with disabilities, and the long-lasting impact of colonialism (Azzoni, 2022; Pinilla-Roncancio, 2015; Taylor, 2016).

The main drawback is the fact that legal recognition is common even when no material transformation occurs. Many Latin American nations have correlated international treaties, such as the Convention on the Rights of Persons with Disabilities (CRPD), with significant developments in the creation of legal and institutional frameworks for the protection and promotion of the rights of disabled people (Leal & Torres, 2024; Meléndez Rojas, 2019; Pinilla-Roncancio & Rodríguez Caicedo, 2022; Rebolledo-Sanhueza & Galaz-Valderrama, 2024). For example, the countries mentioned are Argentina, Bolivia, Brazil, Chile, Colombia, Costa Rica, Ecuador, El Salvador, Guatemala, Haiti, Honduras, Mexico, Nicaragua, Panama, Paraguay, Peru, Dominican Republic, Uruguay, and Venezuela, all of which have some specific laws concerning handicapped individuals (das Mercês Rocha et al., 2020). However, practical results are often not at all comparable to these laws, with an "implementation gap" being a clear indicator of the difference between the existing legal frameworks and their actual use in administration and politics (Martínez Espinoza, 2015; Meléndez Rojas, 2019). This is most noticeable in the field of education, where public policy discourses on equality and socialization for the disabled have changed, and still, the establishment of effective educational models is being rendered unsuccessful by the bad social views and other issues (Lima, et al., 2023; Meléndez Rojas, 2019). The same can be said about the employment right, which, although guaranteed by the CRPD, remains only on paper as far as the actual participation of a significant part of the disabled population in the labor market is concerned (Pinilla-Roncancio & Rodríguez Caicedo, 2022; Pinilla-Roncancio & Gallardo, 2023).

The gap between "rights" and "realities," of course, demonstrates in an obvious way the vast divergence between rights that are granted and those that are experienced. Throughout Latin America, the disabled people dramatically (about 70 million people are affected) need, among other things, access to comprehensive rehabilitation and participation in the community (Pinilla-Roncancio & Gallardo, 2023; Toro-Hernández et al., 2019). Surveys in Peru show that parents of disabled kids are the ones who face the harshest barriers to service access and that they suffer from very negative social attitudes, which are a clear reflection of the extreme and traditional societal views still at play (Aguerre et al., 2019). Moreover, the availability of health and primary health services for disabled persons in Latin America and the Caribbean is minimal, thus slowly killing by 10–20 years the PwD who hence encounter barriers to getting medical care (Gatta et al., 2024; Reichenberger et al., 2024). The shortage of proper programs is primarily due to the very little research on the precise requirements of disabled persons, which ultimately results in weak interventions even in community-based inclusive development initiatives that claim to be rights-promoting (Bachfischer et al., 2023).

Bureaucratization, access difficulties, and systemic exclusion are among the factors that make these problems even worse. The legal systems that classify disability and determine the provision of social services in different Latin American countries may contain contradictions, thus causing (Pinilla-Roncancio, 2015). Legal provisions for adjustments, i.e., for disabled university staff in Canada, are in place; still, disabled teachers struggle to get through the standards made for them and the medicalized views of disability (Waterfield et al., 2018). This suggests that even where legal obligations are clear, bureaucratic obstacles and biases can still prevent full participation. In Latin America, the plight of the indigenous people's socio-economic conditions, along with political violence and historical exclusion, results in the scenario of disability being closely associated with poverty and stigma as a barrier to access health and education (Cleall, 2024; Elias et al., 2008; Lapierre, 2023). The global peripheries of law theory argues that the poorer countries of the Global South are actually more disadvantaged in terms of human rights for people with disabilities due to their limited human and financial resources, thus drawing even more attention to systemic barriers (Chouinard, 2018).

The coloniality of power plays a significant role in the way disability is conceptualized and produced in Latin America (Ferrari, 2020; Gandarilla Salgado et al., 2021; Magallón, 2024). The legal systems have always been colonizing instruments, progressively molding the modern state and altering the concepts of law applied to the native populations (de Mattos et al., 2024; López, 2018). This "legal coloniality" allows for the embedding of Western notions of citizenship and normativity, thus again, not uncommonly, those who do not fit into Eurocentric ideals get excluded or pushed to the margins (Magallón, 2024; Taylor, 2016). An example of this is the concept of "unfitness to stand trial" which, although used in the context of criminal justice systems, has been criticized as being opposite to CRPD's stressing on the need for support given to individuals in exercising legal capacity; it thus shows that colonial legal categories can still lead to the holding of ableist ideas (Mercurio & Sheinbaum Lerner, 2024). The definitions and conceptions of disability mostly circulating in the Latin American region are in a profound interlacing with the coloniality of capability, a crucial feminist decolonial standpoint that not only redefines but also elaborates the analytical categories (Ferrari, 2020). The "rights-bearing subject" in such regimes is often implicitly defined according to prevailing Western, able-bodied, and autonomous ideals, and thus those who do not conform are excluded.

The critiques of rights and inclusion by indigenous people exhibit different perspectives. The indigenous communities of Latin America have been making this claim for centuries, saying that their rights, which are often viewed as collective rights, relationality, and reciprocity, are in no way similar to the Western individualistic rights frameworks (Schmid, 2023; Rice, 2023). The worldviews and cultural practices of the indigenous communities help them to understand and experience disabilities in various ways; thus, they are the ones who challenge the dominant Western concepts (Lovern, 2017; Lapierre, 2023). For instance, the notion of "common" and legal pluralism are the two most essential tools in the process of decolonization in Latin America, which support the self-governance of the community and the ability to manage oneself on a horizontal basis that puts the whole community's well-being above the individualistic legal norms (Nogueira, 2019; Wolkmer & Schumacher Wolkmer, 2022).

Indigenous points of view not only are but also inappropriately characterize disability as such. In the Western model, the disabled individual would not be regarded as a citizen and would not benefit financially from society; thus, disability is equated with the loss of independence and the inability to be productive (Meyers, 2020). The indigenous communities, on the contrary, usually focus on care, responsibility, and communal belonging where these individuals' worth is not entirely dependent on their functional abilities or their capacity to contribute to a capitalist economy (Acevedo et al., 2023; Lapierre, 2023). This is reflected in the cases of women with intellectual disabilities who are still at risk of being violent, but at the same time, they are the ones who look for belongingness and meaningful relationships within their neighborhoods (Pestka & Wendt, 2014). The motherhood aspect of women with disabilities in rural Latin America, especially in indigenous areas, though, aligns with the modern/colonial/Western/urban understanding while also challenging it and thus advocating for the decolonizing practices and knowledge that would recognize the diverse experiences of family and care (Acevedo, et al., 2023; Rodríguez-Garrido & Pino-Morán, 2023; Sanmiquel-Molinero et al., 2023).

In light of these constraints, the power of grassroots disability activism and community-led governance models in Latin America has been recognized as a significant force of change. The organizing of the Indigenous and rural disabled together intends to develop the society, a place where rights will be demanded, but in a manner that reflects the specific culture and community (Pino-Morán et al., 2023). The movements' parallel sides are often mutual help, community care, and informal justice systems which deal with the needs outside the formal, often inaccessible, state structures (Aguerre et al., 2019; Bachfischer et al., 2023; Toro-Hernández et al., 2019). Women and queer-led grassroots movements giving special attention to discriminated and violence-ridden groups within disability communities contribute a lot to these ongoing efforts (Acevedo et al., 2023). Disabled activists in Latin America, particularly in countries like Chile, have practiced revendicative occupational strategies, including conducting in-depth interviews and using social media to claim their rights and challenge their historic marginalization (Pino-Morán et al., 2023). The movements signify a transition period where disabled people start to self-determine their inclusion and justice and thus, avoid the Western rights-based approaches and, thereby, create more equitable and culturally resonant pathways for persons with disabilities in the region.

7.4 Toward Pluriversal Futures of Disability Justice: Self-Determination, Belonging, and Ethical Praxis

The mixing point of Indigenous self-governance and disability in Latin America turns out to be a highly complex issue for the existing policy frameworks, and it also suggests a top-down approach. First of all, the conventional policies are no longer the only position to be adopted in dealing with the matter. Besides, they have a point similar to the existing understanding of disability where the non-Indigenous perceive it as the central aspect of the matter and the Indigenous people as the secondary players, only to be considered for coexistence purposes and, therefore, having no say in the matter. The groups advocating for this shift call it by the use of terms like 'pluriversal' policies and 'relational inclusion and embodied justice states' in terms of the disabilities of the affected people (Lapierre, 2023; Ortega, 2023; Zembylas, 2019).

In Latin America, the indigenous people (Abya Yala and Turtle Island) often have disabilities, and one can say that colonialism, forced assimilation, and poverty are the main influencing factors (Lapierre, 2023). Disability was viewed and dealt with according to the Western medical model, which considers impairment as a defect and consequently treats and cures it as such. This has led to the overlooking of and, indeed, historical marginalization of the various different notions of disability in the context of Indigenous societies (Lovern, 2017; Meekosha, 2011). This situation underlines the need for a decolonization of disability policy, which will support the creation of places for Indigenous scholarship; and non-universal Global North tendencies are among the factors that need to be challenged (Meekosha., 2011; Woods et al., 2018).

Self-governance, Territorial Autonomy, and Disability in Latin America: The self-determination of Indigenous peoples is a fundamental right acknowledged by international law, which grants Indigenous peoples the power to decide their political status and to undertake the development of their economic, social, and cultural lives freely (Velasco & Kline, 2025). In Latin America, this very principle manifests itself in the form of demands for territorial autonomy and self-government, which are considered essential for the proper treatment of disabilities within Indigenous communities according to their respective cultural practices and worldviews (de Freitas et al., 2020; González et al., 2023). The fight for the autonomy of Indigenous peoples in countries like Nicaragua has to cope with strong opposition from the national government, which often results in a hybrid system of governance at the level of subnational units (González, 2016). Even though some countries have gone through constitutional reforms, the problems associated with the lack of a policy catering to urban Indigenous needs still remain, thereby indicating the continuing conflict between the integration of the state and the self-rule of Indigenous people (Ekern, 2011; Horn, 2018).

Disability in Indigenous communities is interpreted and felt through a specific cultural spectrum that differs from the medicalized interpretations that are broadly accepted in the West (Lapierre, 2023). The legal systems in some Latin American countries have started to recognize cultural diversity, yet in practice this is often not the case, resulting in programs that do not mirror the needs of the community as defined by the community (Bachfischer et al., 2023; das Mercês Rocha et al., 2020). Poverty among Indigenous populations with disabilities is compounded by the old dividing lines of ethnicity, race, sex, and physical disability that create unequal distribution of income and limited access to services (Gandelman et al., 2011).

Community-Defined Needs and Priorities on Disability in Latin America: Ground-up should be the starting point for effective disability policy; it should first give recognition to the unique needs and priorities that Indigenous communities have articulated (Bachfischer et al., 2023). Participatory methods are imperative, consisting of the involvement of disabled people in all the steps of policy formulation, from getting the agenda defined to monitoring and assessing the impacts (Colder Carras et al., 2023). Nonetheless, the studies on the particular requirements of people with disabilities in Latin America are few, resulting in the formulation of projects that might not fit the local circumstances well (Bachfischer et al., 2023). It requires a complete reversal of the scenario where the top directed the demarcated territories, forcing the communities unable to express the needs for the basic needs that are supportive of the aspects of self-advocacy (Hiranandani et al., 2014). A case in point is the situation in Chile, where disability rights activists have used their occupational practices to claim their rights in areas that were historically marginalized, and thus the areas of disability rights activism became the areas of reclamation of rights (Pino-Morán et al., 2023).

Decolonizing Participation in Policy-Making on Disability in Latin America: Decolonization of disability policy means not only the denial of the Western paradigm's supremacy but also the guarantee of the Indigenous voices leading the discourse instead of being merely counted (Meekosha, 2011). This transformation requires delegating very few legitimate roles to the participants and proceeding directly to the sharing of power and co-production of the policies (Colder Carras et al., 2023). The International Convention on the Rights of Persons with Disabilities (CRPD) has been a driver behind the acknowledgment of human rights for disabled people all over the world; however, its realization in Latin America is still obstructed and particularly so in the context of Indigenous people's specific realities (Meekosha, 2011; Rebolledo-Sanhueza & Galaz-Valderrama, 2024). The inclusion of the Indigenous viewpoint in the disability-related dialogue is essential because they usually present the conception of body and mind differences that is opposite to the usual Western one and fosters a more comprehensive understanding of the matter (Lovern, 2017). It is imperative that during the whole process, the recognition is not equated with the assimilation into a Western liberal standard, but rather the support of the different cultural identities and practices of Indigenous peoples is held up (Márquez Duarte, 2024).

Reimagining Inclusion Beyond Institutions on Disability in Latin America: Inevitably, inclusion must be re-envisioned beyond just access to institutions, and must also consider relational, spatial, and ecological dimensions that are in harmony with Indigenous worldviews (Litwiller et al., 2023; Trescher & Hauck, 2020). This way of looking at things admits that inclusion is not only concerned with access to the places but also with the genuine acceptance and acknowledgment of being a part of the community (Litwiller et al., 2023).

Inclusion as relational, spatial, and ecological: This viewpoint underlines the individual's close connection with his/her environment, community, and land (Zembylas, 2019). To give an example, relational autonomy points out the fact that the individual is dependent on and has the power to make his/her choice through social relationships and the community's context. The land and environment are at the core of the identity and well-being of Indigenous peoples; therefore, making ecological factors unavoidable in the aspect of inclusion (Merino, 2021; Rodríguez-Garrido & Pino-Morán, 2023).

Land, environment, and embodied justice: The idea behind embodied justice is that disabled people's experiences are directly linked to past and current injustices, one of which is land dispossession and degradation of nature (Merino, 2021; Ortega, 2023). The case of Indigenous women with disabilities living in rural areas illustrates the intersection of motherhood, disability, and rurality, which in turn raises the need for decolonizing practices and knowledge that recognize their special circumstances and bond to the land (Rodríguez-Garrido & Pino-Morán, 2023).

From access to belonging: Transitioning from the area of simply providing access to creating belonging will necessitate changes in the whole system, which will take apart structural barriers and will challenge the prevailing notions of ableism. For the Indigenous people with disabilities, this means not just being there but being actively valued and included in the social fabric and free from the hardships of colonialism and heteropatriarchy (Litwiller et al., 2023).

Toward Pluriversal Disability Policy Frameworks on Disability in Latin America: The advancement of pluriversal disability policy frameworks in Latin America requires the involvement of different knowledge systems, mainly those of Indigenous peoples, to form completely inclusive societies (Ortega, 2023).

Plurinational states and legal pluralism: The idea of plurinationalism, which recognizes the presence of various nations in a single state, is increasingly accepted in Latin America as a way to deal with the issue of cultural diversity and the rights of the Indigenous people (Gustafson, 2009; Merino, 2018). Pluralism in law is often included in this scenario, where the Indigenous customary laws and the state laws are practiced side by side, thus permitting different understandings and approaches to disability within the legally recognized autonomous territories (Assies, 1999). For instance, Bolivia's new constitution lifts plurinationalism and autonomy to a level of official status, mirroring the historical disputes over the rights of the Indigenous people to their lands and citizenship (Gustafson, 2009; García-Domingo et al., 2022).

South–South policy dialogues: Creating dialogues between countries in the Global South can be an effective way to exchange experiences and the best practices in the development of disability policies that are relevant to the local context and do not rely on Northern-centric models (Meekosha, 2011). This partnership can enhance the capacities of the local communities and lead to the development of creative solutions that are adapted to the specific challenges faced by the various communities within Latin America (Hiranandani et al., 2014).

Translating Indigenous worldviews into disability policy without co-optation: One of the main challenges in integrating indigenous knowledge systems into policy is the careful navigation required to avoid co-optation or tokenism, which means (Colder Carras et al., 2023) that Indigenous perspectives are included superficially and without real recognition or power. This implies that Indigenous epistemology would provide the foundation of disability policies and the methods of their implementation, rather than just being lit up through existing Western paradigms (Lovern, 2017). One of the objectives is to come to a situation where Indigenous peoples enjoy complete, prior, and informed consent (FPIC) over policies that impact them (Gil, 2022).

Disability in Latin America: Tensions, Risks, and Ethical Challenges: To attain a share in the Holy Grail of Indigenous self-determination in disability policy, a quagmire of tensions, ethical challenges, and the like must be addressed, without which the issue of just and sustainable outcomes cannot be addressed without careful consideration.

Co-optation, tokenism, and state appropriation: The state of Indigenous movements is riddled with co-optation, whereby the superficial address of the demands of the movements and the appropriation of the state occur, but the changes brought about are not substantial. This could take the form of either superficially participatory policy discussions where the Indigenous representatives are acknowledged but do not have any real power, or the state seizing Indigenous resources and territories by claiming that it is for the purpose of development. The strategy of "you can join us, but only on our terms" adopted by the states always leads to a kind of inclusion that involves being assimilated to the Western liberal standards, which indeed undermines the very essence of self-determination (Colder Carras et al., 2023; Márquez Duarte, 2024).

Internal exclusions within grassroots movements: Grassroots movements can face criticisms from within despite their promotion of human rights of all kinds. In this case, the particular group in question (e.g., women, severely disabled, specific indigenous sub-groups) may receive little support at the margins (Pestka & Wendt, 2014). Intersectionality is critical in this case, as it differentiates the various identities and their disadvantages, which are often layered and thus have to be dealt with within the movements by themselves.

Navigating recognition without assimilation: One of the most significant issues the society is facing today is to come to a consensus on how to worldwide recognize the rights of the indigenous peoples and disabled people without making them into the dominant society's norm (Márquez Duarte, 2024). This task will need very progressive policies that not only allow for diversity but also provide the necessary support for different cultural identities instead of smoothing them into one (Merino, 2018). For example, when the disability issue is considered from an Indigenous perspective, which could see non-normative bodies as just part of the natural diversity rather than a deficit, it runs counter to the Western medical model of disability (Lapierre, 2023; Ortega, 2023). To illustrate, the Chilean National Disability Law of 2010 had self-determination as one of its objectives; however, the law itself is still faced with the problem of how to fit the Western legal concepts with the Indigenous realities during the process of its implementation (Marfull-Jensen & Flanagan, 2015; Yañez & Zúñiga, 2018).

7.5 Conclusion

This chapter is based on the idea that meaningful disability inclusion in Latin America cannot be accomplished only through the importation of top-down rights frameworks but should be the outcome of grassroots struggles, Indigenous worldviews, and the lives of disabled people. The ongoing gaps in implementation, bureaucracy, and the use of legal categories that have their roots in colonialism show the limitations of the universalist and individualistic approaches that are based on the premise of formal recognition and thus are always seeking a transformation of the material aspect in society. By bringing to the fore relationality, collective care, and community belonging, the disability movements coming from the grassroots undermine the dominant notions of autonomy, productivity, and normativity that are deeply rooted in Western policy regimes. The Indigenous viewpoints in particular reconfigure the disability concept from a deficit to that of a part of the community and thus related to land, spirituality, and interdependence. The rethinking of inclusion from below requires not just participation but a redistribution of power, an ethical co-production of knowledge, and a respect for Indigenous self-determination that does not involve either assimilation or co-optation. The pluriversal disability policy frameworks that are based on legal pluralism, territorial autonomy, and South–South exchanges are the ones that present a new approach for justice that is not just proclaimed but actually lived. However, these paths need to be very conscious of the internal inequalities and intersectional exclusions that exist within the movements of the disadvantaged, for they are the main enemies of the progress of disability justice in Latin America. Ultimately, the transformation of inclusion from institutional access to belonging and the change of rights from legal abstractions to embodied, relational, and collective realities will be the determining factors of disability justice in Latin America.

References

Acevedo, M. L., García, X. E., & Moctezuma, A. (2023). Violencias de género hacia mujeres y niñas indígenas con discapacidad en América Latina. *Cahiers franco-latino-américains d'études sur le handicap, 1*, 18. https://doi.org/10.56078/cfla_discapacidad.159

Aguerre, I. M., Riley-Powell, A. R., Weldon, C. T., Pajuelo, M. J., Celis Nacimento, R. A., Puente-Arnao, A., & Paz-Soldan, V. A. (2019). Knocking on doors that Don't open: Experiences of caregivers of children living with disabilities in Iquitos and Lima, Peru. *Disability and Rehabilitation, 41*(21), 2538–2547.

Amorim-Maia, A. T., & Olazabal, M. (2024). Localising the global goal on adaptation through intersectional thinking. *Cities, 154*, 105349. https://doi.org/10.1016/j.cities.2024.105349

Assies, W. (1999). Multi-ethnicity, the state and the law in Latin America. *The Journal of Legal Pluralism and Unofficial Law, 31*(43), 145–158. https://doi.org/10.1080/07329113.1999.10756532

Azzoni, C. (2022). Accessibility and inequality in Latin America. *Regional Science Policy & Practice, 14*(6), 183–184. https://doi.org/10.1111/rsp3.12617

Bachfischer, A., Barbosa, M. C., Rojas, A. A. R., Bechler, R., Schwienhorst-Stich, E. M., Kasang, C., & Parisi, S. (2023). Implementing community based inclusive development for people with disability in Latin America: A mixed methods perspective on prioritized needs and lessons learned. *International Journal for Equity in Health, 22*(1), 147. https://doi.org/10.1186/s12939-023-01966-8

Bixby, L. E. (2024). Intersectional inequalities: How socioeconomic Well-being varies at the intersection of disability, gender, race-ethnicity, and age. *Research in Social Stratification and Mobility, 91*, 100938. https://doi.org/10.1016/j.rssm.2024.100938

Boda, P. A. (2022). Identity making as a colonization process, and the power of disability justice to cultivate intersectional disobedience. *Education Sciences, 12*(7), 462. https://doi.org/10.3390/educsci12070462

Chouinard, V. (2018). Living on the global peripheries of law: Disability human rights law in principle and in practice in the global south. *Laws, 7*(1), 8. https://doi.org/10.3390/laws7010008

Cleall, E. (2024). Disability and postcolonialism. *Postcolonial Studies, 27*(1), 1–16. https://doi.org/10.1080/13688790.2024.2322252

Colder Carras, M., Machin, K., Brown, M., Marttinen, T. L., Maxwell, C., Frampton, B., & Jones, N. (2023). Strengthening review and publication of participatory mental health research to promote empowerment and prevent co-optation. *Psychiatric Services, 74*(2), 166–172. https://doi.org/10.1176/appi.ps.20220085

das Mercês Rocha, R. N., Cortes, F. F., & Nunes, R. (2020). Assessment of individuals with disabilities in Latin America: A comparative study of the legislation. *International Archives of Medicine, 13*. https://doi.org/10.3823/2630

de Freitas, R. C., Araripe, T. A. F., & Moncayo, A. E. N. (2020). A construção da cidadania dos povos indígenas latino americanos a partir do princípio da autodeterminação. *Derecho y Cambio Social, 17*(59). https://doi.org/10.22456/1982-6524.95049

de Mattos, W. P., da Costa Soares, A., Flores, T. A., & Flores, M. D. S. A. (2024). COLONIALISMO JURÍDICO, O GIRO DECOLONIAL EO PRINCÍPIO DA DIGNIDADE DA PESSOA HUMANA NO BRASIL. *ARACÊ, 6*(3), 5534–5552. https://doi.org/10.56238/arev6n3-077

Deerinwater, J., Ho, S., Thompson, V., Wong, A., Erevelles, N., & Morrow, M. (2024). A conversation on disability justice and intersectionality. In *Handbook of disability: Critical thought and social change in a globalizing world* (pp. 503–524). Springer.

Ekern, S. (2011). The production of autonomy: Leadership and community in Mayan Guatemala. *Journal of Latin American Studies, 43*(1), 93–119. https://doi.org/10.1017/S0022216X1000180X

Elias, M. P., Monteiro, L. M. C., & Chaves, C. R. (2008). Accessibility of legal benefits available in Rio de Janeiro for physically handicapped people. *Ciênc Saúde Coletiva, 13*(3), 1041–1050. https://doi.org/10.1590/s1413-81232008000300027

Ferrari, M. B. (2020). Feminismos descoloniales y discapacidad: hacia una conceptualización de la colonialidad de la capacidad. *Nómadas, 52*, 115–131. https://doi.org/10.30578/nomadas.n52a7

Gandarilla Salgado, J. G., García-Bravo, M. H., & Benzi, D. (2021). Two decades of Anibal Quijano's coloniality of power, eurocentrism and Latin America. *Contexto Internacional, 43*, 199–222. https://doi.org/10.1590/s0102-8529.2019430100009

Gandelman, N., Ñopo, H., & Ripani, L. (2011). Traditional excluding forces: A review of the quantitative literature on the economic situation of indigenous peoples, afro-descendants, and people living with disability. *Latin American Politics and Society, 53*(4), 147–179. https://doi.org/10.2139/ssrn.1820909

García-Domingo, M., Fuentes, V., De la Fuente Robles, Y. M., & Muyor, J. (2022). Disability policies and management in Bolivia: Changes and challenges. *Journal of Disability Policy Studies, 33*(1), 55–65. https://doi.org/10.1177/10442073211021987

Gatta, D. R., Rotenberg, S., Allel, K., Reichenberger, V., Banks, L. M., & Kuper, H. (2024). Access to general health care among people with disabilities in Latin America and the Caribbean: A systematic review of quantitative research. *The Lancet Regional Health–Americas, 32*. https://doi.org/10.1016/j.lana.2024.100701

Gil, A. G. (2022). Indigenous peoples, identity and free, prior, and informed consultation in Latin America. In *The Oxford handbook of law and anthropology* (pp. 153–173). Oxford University Press. https://doi.org/10.1093/oxfordhb/9780198840534.001.0001

González, M. (2016). The unmaking of self-determination: Twenty-five years of regional autonomy in N icaragua. *Bulletin of Latin American Research, 35*(3), 306–321. https://doi.org/10.1111/blar.12487

González, M., Funaki, R., A, B. C. y. M., Marimán, J., & Ortiz-T, P. (2023). *Indigenous territorial autonomy and self-government in the diverse Americas* (p. 725). University of Calgary Press. https://library.oapen.org/handle/20.500.12657/63726

Gustafson, B. (2009). Manipulating cartographies: Plurinationalism, autonomy, and indigenous resurgence in Bolivia. *Anthropological Quarterly, 82*(4), 985–1016. https://doi.org/10.1353/anq.0.0094

Hiranandani, V., Kumar, A., & Sonpal, D. (2014). Making community inclusion work for persons with disabilities: Drawing lessons from the field. *Community Development, 45*(2), 151–165. https://doi.org/10.1080/15575330.2014.888090

Horn, P. (2018). Indigenous peoples, the city and inclusive urban development policies in Latin America: Lessons from Bolivia and Ecuador. *Development Policy Review, 36*(4), 483–501. https://doi.org/10.1111/dpr.12234

Lapierre, M. (2023). Disability and Latin American indigenous peoples. *Disability & society, 38*(7), 1276–1280. https://doi.org/10.1080/09687599.2023.2192381

Leal, N. M. O., & Torres, C. P. M. (2024). Una Mirada a la Normatividad Latinoamericana en la Inclusión de Personas con Discapacidad. *Ciencia Latina Revista Científica Multidisciplinar, 8*(2), 4918–4938. https://doi.org/10.37811/cl_rcm.v8i2.10907

Lima, A. P., Lima, V., & Giglio, E. (2023). Education for people with disabilities: Challenges and solutions. *CIVINEDU 2023*, 17.

Litwiller, F., Chesser, S., & Henhawk, D. (2023). Justice as inclusion: A critical conversation about inclusion and belonging. *Leisure/Loisir, 47*(4), 639–658. https://doi.org/10.1080/14927713.2023.2252847

López, P. G. (2018). Colonialidad (jurídica). *Eunomía: Revista en Cultura de la Legalidad, 14*, 205–214. https://doi.org/10.20318/eunomia.2018.4164

Lovern, L. L. (2017). Indigenous perspectives on difference: A case for inclusion. *Journal of literary & cultural disability studies, 11*(3), 303–320. https://doi.org/10.3828/jlcds.2017.24

Magallón, D. M. (2024). La discapacidad en México y nuestra América. Una perspectiva crítica, jurídica y decolonial en construcción en el siglo XXI. *Alternativas en Ciencias Sociales, 1*(1), 47–73.

Marfull-Jensen, M., & Flanagan, T. D. (2015). The 2010 Chilean national disability law: Self-determination in a collectivistic society. *Journal of Disability Policy Studies, 26*(3), 144–152. https://doi.org/10.1177/1044207314533384

Márquez Duarte, F. D. (2024). You can sit with us, but under our terms: The recognition of indigenous self-determination by nation-states throughout the Abya Yala. *Latin American Perspectives, 51*(4), 43–61. https://doi.org/10.1177/0094582X241294082

Martínez Espinoza, M. I. (2015). Reconocimiento sin implementación: Un balance sobre los derechos de los pueblos indígenas en América Latina. *Revista Mexicana de Ciencias Políticas y Sociales, 60*(224), 251–277. https://doi.org/10.1016/S0185-1918(15)30010-6

Meekosha, H. (2011). Decolonising disability: Thinking and acting globally. *Disability & Society, 26*(6), 667–682. https://doi.org/10.1080/09687599.2011.602860

Meléndez Rojas, R. E. (2019). Las políticas públicas en materia de discapacidad en América Latina y su garantía de acceso a una educación inclusiva de calidad. *Actualidades investigativas en educación, 19*(2), 280–307. https://doi.org/10.15517/aie.v19i2.36916

Mercurio, E. N., & Sheinbaum Lerner, D. (2024). Unfitness to stand trial and the social model of disability: Challenges for Latin American criminal justice. *Current Issues in Criminal Justice, 36*(3), 301–317. https://doi.org/10.1080/10345329.2023.2297479

Merino, R. (2018). Reimagining the nation-state: Indigenous peoples and the making of plurinationalism in Latin America. *Leiden Journal of International Law, 31*(4), 773–792. https://doi.org/10.1017/S0922156518000389

Merino, R. (2021). *Socio-legal struggles for indigenous self-determination in Latin America: Reimagining the nation, reinventing the state.* Routledge. https://doi.org/10.4324/9781003129325

Meyers, S. (2020). Rethinking citizenship, self-help, and disability in local context: Solidaridad as disability citizenship in Nicaragua. *Disability Studies Quarterly, 40*(3). https://doi.org/10.18061/dsq.v40i3.6977

Nogueira, T.C. (2019). Legal pluralism: an approach from the new Latin American. *Aspects de droit financier sous-jacents au processus d'impeachment au Br~ sil Financial law aspects underlying the impeachment process in Brazil, 6*(3), 621–645. https://doi.org/10.5380/rinc.v6i3.69579

Ortega, D. C. V. (2023). Tierra de imbunches y ch'uqtas: la dis-capacidad como dispositivo colonial en América Latina y el Caribe. *Brazilian Journal of Latin American Studies, 22*(47), 197–222. https://doi.org/10.11606/issn.1676-6288.prolam.23.213227

Pestka, K., & Wendt, S. (2014). Belonging: Women living with intellectual disabilities and experiences of domestic violence. *Disability & Society, 29*(7), 1031–1045. https://doi.org/10.1080/09687599.2014.902358

Pinilla-Roncancio, M. (2015). Disability and social protection in Latin American countries. *Disability & Society, 30*(7), 1005–1020. https://doi.org/10.1080/09687599.2015.1059316

Pinilla-Roncancio, M., & Gallardo, M. (2023). Inequality in labour market opportunities for people with disabilities: Evidence for six Latin American countries. *Global social policy, 23*(1), 67–91. https://doi.org/10.1177/14680181211070201

Pinilla-Roncancio, M., & Rodríguez Caicedo, N. (2022). Legislation on disability and employment: to what extent are employment rights guaranteed for persons with disabilities? *International journal of environmental research and public health, 19*(9), 5654. https://doi.org/10.3390/ijerph19095654

Pino-Morán, J. A., Zango-Martin, I., Rodríguez-Garrido, P., & Mora-Malo, E. (2023). Reivindicative occupational practices of activist with disabilities. *Cadernos Brasileiros de Terapia Ocupacional, 31*, e3510. https://doi.org/10.1590/2526-8910.ctoao269135102

Polheim, A., Manuel-Navarrete, D., Goebel, J., & Loos, J. (2024). Embodying relationality through immersive sustainability solutions with indigenous communities in the Ecuadorian Amazon. *Sustainability Science, 19*(4), 1445–1457. https://doi.org/10.1007/s11625-024-01523-4

Rebolledo-Sanhueza, J. A., & Galaz-Valderrama, C. (2024). Activismo y discapacidad en Latinoamérica: luchas por el reconocimiento. *Revista Estudos Feministas, 32*(1). https://doi.org/10.1590/1806-9584-2024v32n190769

Reichenberger, V., Corona, A. P., Ramos, V. D., Shakespeare, T., Hameed, S., Penn-Kekana, L., & Kuper, H. (2024). Access to primary healthcare services for adults with disabilities in Latin America and the Caribbean: A review and meta-synthesis of qualitative studies. *Disability and Rehabilitation, 46*(25), 6011–6020. https://doi.org/10.1080/09638288.2024.2320268

Rice, R. (2023). Indigenous Movements in Latin America. In *The Oxford handbook of Latin American social movements* (pp. 354–369). Oxford University Press. https://doi.org/10.1093/oxfordhb/9780190870362.013.18

Riley, T., Meston, T., Cutler, C., Low-Choy, S., McCormack, B. A., Kim, E. J. A., & Vasco, D. (2024). Weaving stories of strength: Ethically integrating indigenous content in teacher education and professional development programmes. *Teaching and Teacher Education, 142*, 104513. https://doi.org/10.1016/j.tate.2024.104513

Rodríguez-Garrido, P., & Pino-Morán, J. A. (2023). Motherhood, disability, and rurality: Descolonising practices and knowledge via the las Quiscas case in Chile. *Gender and Development, 31*(2–3), 361–381. https://doi.org/10.1080/13552074.2023.2254570

Sanmiquel-Molinero, L., Pujol-Tarrés, J., & Montenegro, M. (2023). Latin American perspectives on parenthood and disability: Vulnerability, risk, and social inclusion. *Social Inclusion, 11*(4), 338–349. https://doi.org/10.17645/si.v11i4.7046

Schmid, S. P. (2023). Individual or collective rights? Consequences for the satisfaction with democracy among indigenous peoples in Latin America. *Democratization, 30*(6), 1113–1134. https://doi.org/10.1080/13510347.2023.2213163

Stienstra, D. (2023). (Th) reading rights and justice: Women and girls with disabilities. *Global Society, 37*(3), 354–374. https://doi.org/10.1080/13600826.2022.2146576

Taylor, L. (2016). Decolonizing citizenship: Reflections on the coloniality of power in Argentina. In *Narratives and imaginings of citizenship in Latin America* (pp. 72–86). Routledge. https://doi.org/10.1080/13621025.2013.818375

Toro-Hernández, M. L., Mondragón-Barrera, A., Múnera-Orozco, S., Villa-Torres, L., & Camelo-Castillo, W. (2019). Experiences with rehabilitation and impact on community participation among adults with physical disability in Colombia: Perspectives from stakeholders using a community based research approach. *International Journal for Equity in Health, 18*(1), 18. https://doi.org/10.1186/s12939-019-0923-4

Trescher, H., & Hauck, T. (2020). *Inklusion im kommunalen Raum: Sozialraumentwicklung im Kontext von Behinderung, Flucht und Demenz* (p. 372). transcript Verlag. https://doi.org/10.1515/9783839452677

Velasco, M., & Kline, C. (2025). Indigenous autonomy in Latin America: The impact of the indigenous rights revolution on the study of politics. *Journal of Race, Ethnicity, and Politics, 10*, 1–29. https://doi.org/10.1017/rep.2024.34

Waterfield, B., Beagan, B. B., & Weinberg, M. (2018). Disabled academics: A case study in Canadian universities. *Disability & Society, 33*(3), 327–348. https://doi.org/10.1080/09687599.2017.1411251

Wolkmer, A. C., & Schumacher Wolkmer, M. D. F. (2022). The principle of the common, legal pluralism and decolonization in Latin America. *Law and Critique, 33*(1), 63–87. https://doi.org/10.1007/s10978-021-09285-z

Woods, R., Milton, D., Arnold, L., & Graby, S. (2018). Redefining critical autism studies: A more inclusive interpretation. *Disability & Society, 33*(6), 974–979. https://doi.org/10.1080/09687599.2018.1454380

Yañez, R., & Zúñiga, Y. (2018). The law and occupational justice: Inputs for the understanding of disability in Chile. *Journal of Occupational Science, 25*(4), 520–529. https://doi.org/10.1080/14427591.2018.1522946

Zembylas, M. (2019). A Butlerian perspective on inclusion: The importance of embodied ethics, recognition and relationality in inclusive education. *Cambridge Journal of Education, 49*(6), 727–740. https://doi.org/10.1080/0305764X.2019.1607823

Appendix

Appendix A: Glossary of Terms

Ableism—A system of beliefs and practices that privileges certain bodies and minds while marginalizing disabled people through social, institutional, and cultural norms.

Coloniality—The enduring patterns of power, knowledge, and social relations established during colonialism that persist beyond formal colonial rule (Quijano).

Colonial Medicine—Medical practices introduced during colonial rule that classified, controlled, and disciplined bodies to serve imperial, racial, and economic interests.

Decolonial Disability Studies—An interdisciplinary approach that critiques Eurocentric disability frameworks and centers Global South, Indigenous, and marginalized epistemologies.

Disability Justice—A framework that links disability to broader struggles against racism, colonialism, capitalism, patriarchy, and environmental injustice.

Epistemic Injustice—The systematic devaluation or silencing of certain knowledge systems, particularly Indigenous and disabled ways of knowing.

Grassroots Inclusion—Bottom-up practices of disability inclusion rooted in lived experiences, community knowledge, and local contexts.

Indigenous Worldviews—Holistic systems of knowledge emphasizing relationality, reciprocity, land, spirituality, and collective responsibility.

Legal Pluralism—The coexistence of multiple legal systems, including Indigenous customary law and state law.

Pluriversality—The recognition of multiple coexisting worlds, epistemologies, and ways of being, as opposed to universalism.

S. M. Thomas and R. Veerabathiran, *Disability and Decolonial Thought in Latin America*, SpringerBriefs in Modern Perspectives on Disability Research,
https://doi.org/10.1007/978-981-95-8950-0

Appendix B: Figures and Tables

Figures

Tables

Appendix C: Methodological and Cultural Considerations

This book adopts a qualitative, critical, and decolonial methodological orientation. Rather than relying on extractive or positivist research models, the chapters emphasize:

- Respect for Indigenous knowledge systems and oral traditions.
- Recognition of positionality, power asymmetries, and historical violence.
- Use of interdisciplinary approaches (history, disability studies, anthropology, feminist theory).
- Caution against universalizing disability categories across cultures.
- Ethical emphasis on representation, reciprocity, and epistemic justice.

Culturally, the chapters stress that disability meanings are context-specific, relational, and embedded in land, community, and spirituality. Western diagnostic frameworks are treated critically rather than as neutral tools.

Appendix D: Relevant Frameworks and Policies

International Frameworks

- Convention on the Rights of Persons with Disabilities (CRPD).
- Universal Declaration of Human Rights (UDHR).
- Sustainable Development Goals (SDGs).

Regional and Conceptual Frameworks

- Decolonial Theory (Quijano, Mignolo).
- Disability Justice Framework (Sins Invalid).
- Indigenous Self-Determination and Legal Pluralism.
- Intersectionality (Race, Gender, Disability, Class).

Critical Observations

While international frameworks provide formal recognition, the chapters highlight persistent implementation gaps, cultural misalignment, and the risk of policy co-optation when Indigenous and grassroots voices are excluded.

Appendix E: Statistical Insights

Although this book is not a quantitative study, existing regional data contextualize the arguments presented:

- Approximately 80% of the global disabled population lives in the Global South.
- Latin America accounts for nearly 70 million persons with disabilities.
- Disabled Indigenous populations experience higher poverty, lower education access, and reduced healthcare coverage.
- Life expectancy for persons with disabilities in parts of Latin America is 10–20 years shorter due to systemic barriers.
- Legal ratification of disability rights does not equate to material inclusion, particularly in rural and Indigenous regions.

These statistics are used analytically, not empirically, to demonstrate structural inequality rather than to define disability experiences numerically.